The Future of Nursing: Advancing Nursing Education and Practice through Technology

Editor

JONI TORNWALL

NURSING CLINICS
OF NORTH AMERICA

www.nursing.theclinics.com

Consulting Editor
BENJAMIN SMALLHEER

December 2022 • Volume 57 • Number 4

ELSEVIER

1600 John F. Kennedy Boulevard ● Suite 1800 ● Philadelphia, Pennsylvania, 19103-2899

http://www.theclinics.com

NURSING CLINICS OF NORTH AMERICA Volume 57, Number 4
December 2022 ISSN 0029-6465, ISBN-13: 978-0-323-98743-1

Editor: Kerry Holland
Developmental Editor: Axell Ivan Jade M. Purificacion

Nursing Clinics of North America (ISSN 0029-6465) is published quarterly by Elsevier Inc., 360 Park Avenue South, New York, NY 10010-1710. Months of issue are March, June, September, and December. Periodicals postage paid at New York, NY and additional mailing offices. Subscription price per year is, $163.00 (US individuals), $689.00 (US institutions), $275.00 (international individuals), $710.00 (international institutions), $231.00 (Canadian individuals), $710.00 (Canadian institutions), $100.00 (US and Canadian students), and $135.00 (international students). To receive student/resident rate, orders must be accompanied by name of affiliated institution, date of term, and the signature of program/residency coordinator on institution letterhead. Orders will be billed at individual rate until proof of status is received. Foreign air speed delivery is included in all *Clinics* subscription prices. All prices are subject to change without notice. **POSTMASTER:** Send address changes to *Nursing Clinics*, Elsevier Health Sciences Division, Subscription Customer Service, 3251 Riverport Lane, Maryland Heights, MO 63043. **Customer Service: Telephone: 1-800-654-2452** (U.S. and Canada); **1-314-447-8871 (outside U.S. and Canada). Fax: 1-314-447-8029.** E-mail: journalscustomerservice-usa@elsevier.com (for print support) and journalsonlinesupport-usa@elsevier.com (for online support).

Nursing Clinics of North America is covered in *EMBASE/Excerpta Medica, MEDLINE/PubMed (Index Medicus), Social Sciences Citation Index, Current Contents, ASCA, Cumulative Index to Nursing, RNdex Top 100,* and Allied Health Literature and International Nursing Index (INI).

Contributors

CONSULTING EDITOR

BENJAMIN SMALLHEER, PhD, RN, ACNP-BC, FNP-BC, CCRN, CNE
Associate Clinical Professor, School of Nursing, Duke University, Durham, North Carolina

EDITOR

JONI TORNWALL, PhD, RN
Associate Professor of Clinical Nursing, Co-Director of the Academy for Teaching Innovation, Excellence, and Scholarship, The Ohio State University College of Nursing, Columbus, Ohio

AUTHORS

GERRY ALTMILLER, EdD, APRN, ACNS-BC, ANEF, FAAN
Professor of Nursing, The College of New Jersey, School of Nursing and Health Sciences, Nursing Education and Professional Development, Ewing, New Jersey

ELIZABETH ANNE CROOKS, DNP, RN, CNE
Instructor, School of Nursing, University of Alabama at Birmingham, Birmingham, Alabama

HEIDI BOBEK, DNP, APRN-CNP
FNP Specialty Track Director, Assistant Professor of Clinical Practice, Family Nurse Practitioner, The Ohio State University College of Nursing, Columbus, Ohio

STEPHANIE BURLINGAME, RN, BSN
Skills and Simulation Faculty, Technology Learning Complex, Ohio State University College of Nursing Columbus, Columbus, Ohio

HOLLY CHESNICK, MS, RN, NE-BC
Director of Nursing, Ambulatory Services, Wexner Medical Center at The Ohio State University; Formerly Nurse Manager, Tower 5 Cardiology Inpatient Unit, East Hospital, Wexner Medical Center at The Ohio State University, Columbus, Ohio

RITA F. D'AOUST, PhD, ANP-BC, CNE, FAANP, FAAN
Associate Dean for Teaching and Learning, Johns Hopkins School of Nursing, Baltimore, Maryland

MIRANDA BERTIE DICKERSON, MS, RN, CHSE
Undergraduate Simulation Coordinator, Technology Learning Complex, Instructor of Clinical Practice, Ohio State University College of Nursing Columbus, Columbus, Ohio

ELIZABETH BURGESS DOWDELL, PhD, RN, AFN-C, FAAN
Professor, Coordinator, Undergraduate Research, Villanova University, M. Louise Fitzpatrick College of Nursing, Philadelphia, Pennsylvania

EDITH A. HARTER, BSN, RN, CHSE
Skills and Simulation Faculty, Technology Learning Complex, Ohio State University
College of Nursing Columbus, Columbus, Ohio

ELIZABETH HUTSON, PhD, APRN-CNP, PMHNP-BC
Associate Professor, Texas Tech University Health Sciences Center, School of Nursing,
Lubbock, Texas

AMY JACKSON, MS, RN, CNL, NE-BC
Nurse Manager, Ambulatory Services, Wexner Medical Center at The Ohio State
University; Formerly Nurse Manager, Tower 7 Medical-Surgical Inpatient Unit,
East Hospital, Wexner Medical Center at The Ohio State University, Columbus,
Ohio

ELISA C. JANG, DNP, MS, RN, CNS, EBP-C
Professional Development Specialist, Leadership Institute, Center for Nursing Excellence
& Innovation, UCSF Health, San Francisco, California

STEPHANIE JUSTICE, DNP, RN, CHSE
Assistant Professor of Clinical Nursing, Ohio State University College of Nursing
Columbus, Columbus, Ohio

LAURA STINNETTE LUCAS, DNP, APRN-CNS, RNC-OB, C-EFM
Assistant Professor, Associate Director of MSN (Entry into Practice) Program, Johns
Hopkins School of Nursing, Baltimore, Maryland

JERI A. MILSTEAD, PhD, RN
Senior Nurse Consultant, Dublin, Ohio

**STACEY A. MITCHELL, DNP, MBA, MEd, RN, AFN-C, SANE-A, SANE-P, DF-AFN,
FAAN**
Clinical Professor, Program Coordinator, Master of Science in Nursing, Forensic Nursing
Track, Director, Center of Excellence in Forensic Nursing, Texas A&M University College
of Nursing, College Station, Texas

YOLANDA M. NELSON, EdD, MSN-Ed, RN-BC
Assistant Professor, School of Nursing and Health Sciences, Trenton Hall, Ewing,
New Jersey

SUNNY BIDDLE NETHERS, MSN, RN
Central Ohio Technical College Nursing Faculty, Newark; Genesis Healthcare System,
Zanesville, Ohio

DÓNAL P. O'MATHÚNA, PhD
Associate Professor, College of Nursing, and Center for Bioethics and Medical
Humanities, The Ohio State University, Columbus, Ohio

LORAINE HOPKINS PEPE, PhD, RN, NPD-BC, CCRN-K
Director, Nursing Education and Professional Development, Jefferson-Einstein
Healthcare Network, Philadelphia, Pennsylvania

LISA ROHRIG, MS, RN, CHSE, CHSOS
Director, Technology Learning Complex, Clinical Instructor of Practice, Ohio State
University College of Nursing Columbus, Columbus, Ohio

LINDA A. ROUSSEL, PhD, RN, NEA-BC, CNL
Department of Graduate Studies, Clinical Professor, School of Nursing, UT Houston Cizik School of Nursing, Houston, Texas

SARAH RUSNAK, MS, RD, LD
Clinical Instructor, School of Health and Rehabilitation Sciences, The Ohio State University College of Medicine, Columbus, Ohio

JOANNE SILBERT-FLAGG, DNP, CPNP, IBCLC, CNE, FAAN
Associate Professor, Director of MSN (Entry into Practice) Program, Johns Hopkins School of Nursing, Baltimore, Maryland

PATRICIA M. SPECK, DNSC, FNP-BC, AFN-C, DF-IAFN, FAAFS, DF-AFN, FAAN
Professor, Coordinator, Advanced Forensic Nursing, Department of Family, Community, & Health Systems, UAB | The University of Alabama at Birmingham School of Nursing, Birmingham, Alabama

JONI TORNWALL, PhD, RN
Associate Clinical Professor, Director for Assessment and Evaluation, Co-Director of the Academy for Teaching Innovation, Excellence, and Scholarship, The Ohio State University College of Nursing, Columbus, Ohio

TODD E. TUSSING, DNP, RN, CENP, NEA-BC
Assistant Clinical Professor, College of Nursing, The Ohio State University; formerly Administrative Director for Nursing and Patient Care Services, East Hospital, Wexner Medical Center at The Ohio State University, Columbus, Ohio

NANCY P. WINGO, PhD, MA
Associate Professor, School of Nursing, University of Alabama at Birmingham, Birmingham, Alabama

Contents

> Professional burnout is a significant occupational hazard resulting in lower
> job commitment, poor patient outcomes, reduced performance, lower job
> satisfaction, and frequent absenteeism. Models exist that provide guid-
> ance in addressing burnout, improving resiliency, and well-being.
> Advancing evidence-based, multidisciplinary solutions to improve patient
> care by caring for the caregiver is the cornerstone to increasing resiliency,
> well-being, empathy, and gratitude. Developing resilience in health care in-
> cludes a wide array of technological methods to facilitate well-being. Dig-
> ital journaling, mood tracking, meditation apps, habit tracking, lifestyle
> apps, and wearable technology are strategies to deal with stress and
> compassion fatigue.

> Continuing education is essential for professional nurses to meet the chal-
> lenges of today's dynamic health care environment. Nursing professional
> development practitioners need to stay abreast of the latest methods
> and best practices in development, delivery, and evaluation of continuing
> education needs. Competency-based continuing education programs are
> based on principles of adult learning and contribute to a culture of auton-
> omy and empowerment. The use of educational technology and collabo-
> ration among emerging clinical roles facilitates opportunities for
> professional nurses to stay engaged in lifelong learning.

> This article examines the concept of telepresence and the use of video
> chat platforms to facilitate family and nurse presence in hospital settings.
> Ethical, technical, and logistical challenges for using video chat platforms
> at the bedside are addressed. In addition, the Community of Inquiry
> model is used to explore how human presence is facilitated in
> distance-accessible nursing education. Special focus is on the use of
> technology to meet the challenges of presence during virtual nursing
> instruction.

Student response systems (SRSs) can be used in online nursing courses to promote student engagement with the course content, their classmates, and the instructor. An overview of the challenges and opportunities of SRSs in online nursing education are described, and examples of implementation of an SRS in an online, synchronous nursing course are provided. Recommendations and best practices for using SRSs in nursing education are summarized.

Despite the unprecedented obstacles created by the COVID-19 pandemic, nursing professional development practitioners and nurse educators successfully harnessed educational technology to disseminate an extraordinary amount of vital information needed to provide care to a society in crisis. The agile adoption of educational technology allowed rapid access and dissemination of information that carried institutions through the uncharted waters of the pandemic and created a roadmap for mass education techniques to guide not only future disaster preparedness and crisis intervention but also application of nursing education in all arenas.

The need to increase diversity in the profession of nursing requires innovative approaches to recruit, retain, and graduate nurses from diverse racial populations. Mentorship has proven to be an effective retention and success strategy for nursing students. This article describes best practices for mentoring nursing students of color and aims to increase awareness of the impact of mentorship and its role in increasing diversity within the profession of nursing. The role technology plays in the facilitation of flexible and effective mentorship programs is explored.

Nurse educators and students are partners in co-creation of a classroom culture of assessment for learning rather than assessment of learning. Three essential sources of feedback—instructor feedback, peer feedback, and self-reflection—contribute to development of metacognitive skills necessary for nursing practice. Triangulation of feedback from multiple sources develops skills in peer evaluation, professional accountability, emotional regulation, and lifelong learning. Feedback processes are supported by creative use of learning technologies such as learning management systems, survey tools, videography using institutional equipment or students' personal devices, social annotation strategies and applications, and audience response systems.

Physical assessment courses for nurses typically include a didactic education component and a physical skills laboratory for hands-on practice. Skills instruction focuses on a head-to-toe assessment of body systems, including inspection, palpation, percussion, and auscultation. Comparable learning outcomes can be achieved in both online and traditional classrooms. Telehealth education needs to be included in physical assessment instruction as telehealth services expand to provide greater access to health care. This article provides strategies for incorporating education into online physical assessment courses for nurses and suggests online resources for effective telehealth integration into clinical practice.

Humanity is facing an increasing threat to life and property due to an increase in disasters. Disasters occur with little warning and can last for hours or months. Current literature reveals that most nurses are not prepared for a disaster in their community. Continual readiness requires the engagement of staff and nursing students in disaster plan development, review, and implementation. Development of educational training programs that are ongoing, easily accessible, engaging, and realistic is best for skills and competency acquisition. Technology, such as virtual simulation, shows great potential to prepare health care professionals and should be incorporated into disaster preparedness plans.

Health care ethics education has focused on the four principles approach. Although relevant and important, this dimension is insufficient on its own. Emotional, cultural, spiritual, and relational aspects of ethics must also be addressed. Ethics cases are important in ethics education but should include everyday ethics scenarios that can be messy and emotional. Such situations occur regularly in nursing practice, making microethics particularly relevant to nurses. Art, songs, film, and literature provide stories that allow exploration of everyday ethics. Technology can facilitate this and promote ethics comportment, but more work is needed to demonstrate how best to do this.

This article addresses the relationship of governmental laws and regulations and private sector policies to nurse practice. Integration of the policy process in nurse education curricula is discussed in relationship to the potential to effect sustainable, equitable policy change and prepare nurses who are ready to assume leadership roles. Nurse input in the selection, use, and evaluation of technology in education, practice, and policy is framed within the leadership role of the basic and advanced nurse.

NURSING CLINICS

SERIES OF RELATED INTEREST

Advances in Family Practice Nursing
www.advancesinfamilypracticenursing.com

THE CLINICS ARE AVAILABLE ONLINE!
Access your subscription at:
www.theclinics.com

FORTHCOMING ISSUES

March 2023
COVID-19 and Pandemic Preparedness:
Lessons Learned and Next Steps
Kelly A. Wolgast, Editor

June 2023
Substance Use and Abuse
Linda Stone, Editor

September 2023
Updates and Advances in Cardiovascular
Nursing
Leslie L. Davis, Editor

RECENT ISSUES

September 2022
Vulnerable Populations
Angela Richard-Eaglin, Editor

June 2022
Nursing Leadership in Long-Term Care
Melodee Harris, Ann Kolanowski, and
Sherry Greenberg, Editors

March 2022
Burnout in Nursing: Causes, Management,
and Future Directions
George A. Zangaro, Dorothy Dulko, Debra
Sullivan, Editors

SERIES OF RELATED INTEREST

Advances in Family Practice Nursing
www.advancesinfamilypracticenursing.com

THE CLINICS ARE AVAILABLE ONLINE!
Access your subscription at:
www.theclinics.org

Preface

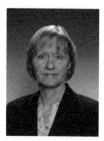

Joni Tornwall, PhD, RN
Editor

Technology played a pivotal role in our ability as nurses and educators to adapt to sudden disruptions in familiar paradigms during the COVID-19 pandemic. Our agile response was supported in part by innovative approaches to using technology to maintain continuity in academic and professional education, care for patients via telehealth, keep patients connected with their loved ones, and sustain our own mental health and resilience. Many of the rapid changes that we experienced during the pandemic catalyzed innovations and shifts in thinking about the way we will practice and teach nursing in the future and are covered in this issue of *Nursing Clinics of North America*. They include the following:

- Active involvement of nurses in policy creation to keep up with rapid changes in how technology affects education and practice
- Better education related to telehealth as an effective and flexible way to deliver health care
- Health and wellness apps with social networking features to support patient care, professional development, and resilience of the health care workforce
- Approaches to disaster preparedness that leverage mobile technology and virtual simulations

Proficiency in the use of technology to support health care processes and positive patient outcomes is an essential nursing competency,[1] and threading technology instruction through nurse education curricula is crucial in the preparation of practice-ready nurses. Throughout this issue, the integral role of technology in education and practice is made apparent through specific examples from the classroom, entry-level nursing contexts, and advanced and specialty practice settings. The authors describe technology-based strategies to engage students in clinical reasoning, teach new nurses working on a med-surg unit to operate medical equipment, and provide practical experience for forensic nurses in completing an electronic death certificate.

Skilled instructional designers and content experts enhance student engagement in nursing education by using technology to facilitate connections to experts, mentors, peers, and instructional resources, which is crucial for students who might otherwise

https://doi.org/10.1016/j.cnur.2022.09.001
0029-6465/22/© 2022 Published by Elsevier Inc.
nursing.theclinics.com

lack educational access and support. Technology makes multimodal approaches to learning possible through multiple types of media and sensory inputs and allows learners to produce observable, measurable responses to assessments that demonstrate knowledge and competency. Case-based stories, educational games, student-driven instruction, peer-to-peer teaching and feedback, and collaborative decision making in ambiguous situations are strategies described in this issue that are readily implemented through thoughtfully selected technology.

Nurse educators in academic and practice settings need to stay up to date in a constantly evolving landscape of learning technologies and know how to mitigate potential barriers, such as cost and access in technology implementation. Investments in technology infrastructure, instructional design experts, and faculty development are critical to maximizing the power of technology in the future of nursing practice and education. This issue of *Nursing Clinics of North America* is designed to inform decisions by nurses about delivery of patient care and nurse education and inspire them to express their own creativity and innovation by taking advantage of the benefits technology has to offer to education and practice now and in the future.

Joni Tornwall, PhD, RN
The Ohio State University College of Nursing
1585 Neil Avenue
Columbus, OH 43210, USA

E-mail address:
tornwall.2@osu.edu

REFERENCE

1. American Association of Colleges of Nursing (AACN). The essentials: core competencies for professional nursing education. Washington, DC: AACN; 2021. Available at: https://www.aacnnursing.org/Portals/42/AcademicNursing/pdf/Essentials-2021.pdf. Accessed March 16, 2022.

On-the-Go Strategies to Enhance Resilience and Self-Care

Using Technology to Create Healthy Work Cultures

Linda A. Roussel, PhD, RN, NEA-BC, CNL*

KEYWORDS

- Gamification • Healthy work environments • Mobile applications
- Organizational culture • Professional burnout • Resilience • Self-care • Well-being

KEY POINTS

- Health care delivery during the coronavirus disease outbreak heralded increasing challenges for the global nursing workforce, placing them at a higher risk for occupational burnout and turnover.
- Creating a healthy work environment and joy in work enables nurses to provide the highest standards of compassionate patient care as well as renew meaningful work and job satisfaction.
- Health care systems that regularly assess burnout and nurses' well-being can more deftly adjust salaries, bonus cycles, grow well-being programs, and expand professional development practices to anticipate and eliminate nurse attrition.
- There are a variety of technological strategies available that include healthy ways to deal with stress and compassion fatigue, as well as lifestyle apps and wearables that are essential to daily self-care practices.

BACKGROUND

The 2019 World Happiness Report notes that negative feelings, including worry, sadness, and anger, have been rising around the world, up by 27% from 2010 to 2018.[1] There are several factors that contribute to this increased negativity, including ways we communicate and connect through social media, use of big data, and lack of meaningful interaction through community and work. Goh and colleagues[2] reported that stressful jobs contribute to 120,000 deaths each year and cost US businesses

Department of Graduate Studies, School of Nursing, UT Houston Cizik School of Nursing, 6901 Bertner Avenue, Suite 648, Houston, TX 77030, USA
* 1415 Denise Drive, New Braunfels, TX 78130.
E-mail address: Linda.A.Roussel@uth.tmc.edu

Nurs Clin N Am 57 (2022) 501–512
https://doi.org/10.1016/j.cnur.2022.06.002
0029-6465/22/© 2022 Elsevier Inc. All rights reserved.

nursing.theclinics.com

up to $190 billion in health care costs. These stressors predominantly impact minorities with low levels of education who often work in unhealthy environments that can shorten lifespans. The researchers looked at 228 studies examining how 10 workplace stressors affect a person's health and used an algorithm to break down the results based on ethnicity. Workplace stressors had the largest impact on non-Hispanic black men with less than 12 years of education, whose life expectancy decreased about 1.7 years. Non-Hispanic white women with more than 17 years of education were the least impacted, losing 0.3 years from their lives due to workplace stressors.[2]

The Future of Nursing Campaign for Action[3] report describes the importance of nurses' helping people live their healthiest lives, an essential role of nursing. Conversely, the health and well-being of nurses influences the quality, safety, and cost of the care they provide, as well as the organizations and systems of care. The coronavirus disease (COVID-19) has starkly revealed the challenges nurses face every day and has added significant new challenges.[3] Ongoing stress, anxiety, and compassion fatigue have significant implications for frontline staff. In the United States, clinical professionals describe suffering from stress and burnout in the workplace, with 35% to 54% affecting nurses and physicians, and 45% to 60% impacting medical students and residents.[4] It is estimated that there are $4.6 billion in societal costs attributable to burnout in the United States each year.[4] The workplace can create physical, mental, emotional, and ethical challenges, including physical or verbal assault; high physical demands; management of the complex needs of multiple patients; necessary emotional conversations with patients and families; overwhelming social and ethical issues; and discrimination from colleagues and patients.[4]

The COVID-19 pandemic heralded greater stress in the workplace with the onset of "The Great Resignation," attributed to ongoing tension and anxiety in the job. In an interview with Bloomberg,[5] Anthony Klotz, an organizational psychologist and professor at Texas A&M University, introduced the term the "Great Resignation" in May 2021 to describe the wave of people quitting their jobs due to the ongoing coronavirus pandemic. This has led employees to rethink where, how, and why they work. For example, in November 2021, a record 4.5 million workers left their jobs, according to the Labor Department's latest Job Openings and Labor Turnover report.[6,7] The Great Resignation has inspired other terms to describe the work revolution, including "The Great Reimagination," "The Great Reset," and "The Great Realization."[6] These descriptive terms provide a perspective on how managers and the workforce are reexamining the role of work in their personal lives. However, they often miss the broader consequences of this quitting wave and what it means for the individual worker. That is, seeking more from work, such as greater autonomy and a more meaningful personal life, before making the decision to resign. Employees are examining the importance of rethinking work for greater control, confidence, competence, and meaning in our job roles.[6,7]

A wide array of technological approaches to facilitating well-being is readily available that can offer creative and imaginative ways to gain more self-determination at all levels of staff engagement. Frameworks are available for assessing burnout and building and sustaining healthy work environments (HWE) and joy in work, and the frameworks underpin evidence-based strategies to enhance resilience and well-being in the workplace. Healthy approaches to dealing with stress, burnout, and compassion fatigue include digital journaling, meditation apps, habit tracking, lifestyle apps, wearable technology, and e-mentoring programs.

Assessing Burnout

Health care systems are concerned about their employees' well-being and satisfaction with work and their work environment. Assessing how employees are faring in their work environment is critical to real and sustained improvement and change. Although several instruments measuring health care provider (HCP) well-being have established reliability and validity, they are not all equally realistic for use by organizations interested in local assessment and quality improvement initiatives. Dyrbye and colleagues[8] provide a list of considerations for individuals challenged with assessing HCP well-being in their systems to guide them in choosing relevant measurement instruments. This decision depends on the dimensions of well-being that are most critical to stakeholders as well as the survey instrument's characteristics. For example, instrument characteristics could include respondent and organizational burden, sensitivity to change, psychometric support, and the tool's application.[8] The Maslach Burnout Inventory-Human Services Survey for Medical Personnel (MBI-HSS [MP]) is the most frequently employed instrument to measure burnout in HCPs.[8] Specifically, the MBI-HSS [MP] has three domains: emotional exhaustion, depersonalization, and low sense of personal accomplishment.

Measuring burnout can also be accomplished by using the Oldenburg Burnout Inventory (OBI) and the Copenhagen Burnout Inventory (CBI).[7] Domains included in the OBI are physical, cognitive, and affective exhaustion, and disengagement from work. Personal (physical and psychological fatigue and exhaustion), work (physical and psychological fatigue and exhaustion related to work), and client-related (or a similar term, such as patient, student, and so forth) burnout are domains included in the CBI. Using a single-item question—for example, the Physician Worklife Study— has also been a choice of health systems and investigators.[8] Using reliable and valid instruments to measure burnout can be the first step in selecting unique, tailored strategies to improve individual workers' well-being and HWE.

FRAMEWORKS AND MODELS

Armed with valid assessments of burnout, managers can lead teams in addressing workplace tension and employee well-being. Conceptual frameworks and models provide context for aligning evidence-based strategies to health care workplace settings and employee needs. Two examples of robust models are described later.

Healthy Work Environments Standards

Creating a HWE enables nurses to provide the highest standards of compassionate patient care while being fulfilled at work. The American Association of Critical Care Nurses (AACN)[9] data consistently describe nursing units that are implementing HWE standards as outperforming those that have not incorporated the standards. The six HWE standards include:

- Skilled communication
- True collaboration
- Effective decision-making
- Appropriate staffing
- Meaningful recognition
- Authentic leadership

The AACN's six essential standards provide evidence-based guidelines for providing high-quality, compassionate patient care while finding fulfillment at work.[9] The healthiest work environments are those that integrate all six standards. After implementing the HWE standards, managers and colleagues noted improvement in staff and patient outcomes in the overall health of the work environment, better nurse staffing and retention, less moral distress, and lower rates of workplace violence.[9]

Specifically, nurses reported that when staffing was appropriate more than 75% of the time, they were able to accomplish more, reports of moral distress were less frequent, overall job satisfaction improved, and the intention to leave their position decreased. Survey respondents reported that when their workplaces had a zero tolerance for abuse policy, there were fewer negative incidents.[9]

Joy in Work

With increasing demands on time, resources, and energy, confounded by poorly designed systems of daily work and an increase in staff turnover, it makes sense that health care professionals would experience burnout at alarmingly high rates.[10] Burnout leads to lower levels of staff engagement, productivity, poorer patient experiences, and an increased risk of workplace accidents. Lower levels of staff engagement are linked to lower-quality patient care and safety, and increased nurse burnout, which limits providers' empathy, an essential element component of effective and person-centered care.[10]

What can health care leaders do to address this epidemic of burnout? The IHI[10] believes an important part of the solution is to focus on renewing joy in the health care workforce. An IHI[10] framework for improving joy in work serves as a guide for health care organizations to engage in a participative process where leaders ask colleagues at all levels of the organization what brings them joy. By asking what matters, leaders encourage colleagues to share their perspectives, and in turn, managers can better understand the barriers to joy in work and co-create meaningful, highly valued strategies to address these issues. Each step serves as the foundation for the steps that follow. First, leaders engage colleagues to identify what matters to them in their work. Step 1 is to start the conversation with questions such as the following:

- What makes for a good day for you?
- What makes you proud to work here?
- When we are at our best, what does that look like?

This can set the context for asking what gets in the way of a good day or what makes for a bad day.

The second step involves leaders identifying the processes, issues, or circumstances that are impediments to what matters—the barriers that get in the way of meeting professional, social, and psychological needs. Leaders can facilitate identifying unique local impediments to joy in work and begin to address the psychological needs of the workforce. This offers everyone a chance to give input on which barriers to address, build camaraderie by working together to remove roadblocks, and practice equity in respecting all voices.

In the third step, multidisciplinary teams come together in partnership to share responsibility for removing these impediments, focusing on critical components and improving and sustaining joy. Step 4 involves leaders and staff working together to accelerate improvement and create a more joyful and productive place to work through improvement science.[10]

Frameworks and models can help managers connect concepts and factors that may aid in aligning the best evidence-based practices to address burnout and caregiver well-being. By using a framework to acknowledge and assess stressful work environments, nurse leaders can make available a variety of ways to deal with stress and compassion fatigue. Providing an array of technology-supported strategies to facilitate healthy work-life balance can promote HWE where HCPs can find meaning in their work.

STRATEGIES TO ENHANCE RESILIENCE AND SELF-CARE

Armed with an understanding of the local and global problems that burnout represents, tools to assess burnout, and frameworks or models to contextualize HWE, managers can holistically consider a variety of technological methods to mitigate burnout. Digital journaling, meditation apps, and habit tracking are examples of healthy ways to encourage employees to deal with stress and compassion fatigue and build a resilient workforce. Lifestyle apps and wearables also play an important role in daily self-care practices.

Digital Journaling

Digital journaling provides an opportunity for reflection in real time. Ohren and colleagues[11] found that digital journaling largely afforded the same benefits as writing by hand, with no sacrifice of emotional expression. For example, two-thirds of the study participants agreed or strongly agreed with the statement, "My typewritten entries this month expressed my innermost thoughts and feelings."[11] Participants found the digital format easy to use and an efficient way of capturing their thoughts.[11] This is particularly relevant as most people have their devices readily available, in contrast to a paper journal or physical notebook (often tucked away on a bedside table). Journaling apps that can be synchronized across platforms allow users to quickly type entries on the device they have handy when inspiration strikes.

Digital journaling tools usually contain a range of features that create a richer experience for the user, such as support for voice dictation and automatic recording of date, time, location, and weather details. Most of these tools also allow for the integration of media, such as photos and graphics, into digital journal entries. Borkin[12] describes digital journaling as most valuable in facilitating creative self-expression, particularly being able to use photos, images, or coloring to enhance the creative process. Journal apps are available with features that will appeal to a wide variety of users.[13] For example, Day One[14] is designed for Mac and iOS users, Momento[15] for social media power users, and Daylio[16] for nonwriters.[13]

The various digital journal apps have features that enhance each user's unique needs and self-care practices. For example, Day One allows users to create journal entries with just one click on the Mac from the menu bar, use templates to make journaling easier, and automatically add metadata, such as location, motion activity, weather, music, and step count. Optional prompts are provided for those who are not sure what to journal about. Users can tag entries with hashtags, insert photos and videos, and set up a password to protect their journal entries. The user can select the free version or pay for additional features.[14]

Momento may be a good choice for regular participants on social media sites, such as Facebook, Twitter, Instagram, or Medium.[15] For regular social media users, Momento can help aggregate shared posts and interactions from the various sites into one place, assisting with a digital archive of online interactions. Further, Momento supports 11 feeds, such as Uber trip histories, Spotify saved tracks, and YouTube videos, in addition to the "traditional" creation of new journal entries in a typical journaling app. Momento remembers where users have been and links to past journal entries. The digital writer can group separate entries (or "moments") into "events." For example, Instagram photos tagged for a special event (wedding, family reunion, graduation, high school reunion) could be put together. Momento also has preset reminders, such as "what did you think about the art class?" at 1 PM and "how would you describe your day?" at 9 PM that prompt journaling and help overcome writer's block.[15]

Digital journaling should consider the writer's communication and learning styles. For example, for those who prefer visuals, *Daylio* captures an individual's mood and activities for each day and eliminates writing or typing entirely for those who prefer to journal through images and icons (adding supplementary notes is optional). The user records their mood by selecting one of five smiley-face icons. Additional icons are available to illustrate what the user accomplished that day (eg, running, visiting a museum, visiting a friend), along with customized mood and activity icons. Capturing a person's moods, activities, and the day's events is efficient and takes only seconds, with the details coming together to illustrate a well-rounded picture of a day that can be shared with friends and family. Along with typical digital journaling features, such as reminders and goal setting, *Daylio* offers a detailed dashboard that aggregates a monthly mood chart, including activity counts and average daily moods. Through tracking, *Daylio* illustrates patterns in the "Often together" section, which demonstrates "usual" perceptions while engaging in certain activities (eg, when the user's mood is "good," they are usually spending time with family and friends).[16]

Digital journaling, similar to traditional journaling, provides opportunities for reflection and mindfulness. Digital journaling can reduce stress by serving as an escape or emotional release of negative thoughts and feelings, improve physical health, support problem-solving, and assist with putting daily life experiences into perspective.[17] Digital journaling offers a technological strategy that can be accessed anywhere, any time, and in a variety of online formats, providing people who prefer not to write with viable options to gain the benefits of self-reflection in reducing stress and burnout and increasing well-being.[11,17]

Meditation Apps

Meditation, an excellent strategy to reflect, refocus, and achieve centeredness, can be unusually difficult to learn and master. Meditation apps act as technology-based guides and can facilitate meditation by making it easier and more intuitive for first-time meditators or seasoned pros who have had lapses in their meditation practice.[18] One benefit of meditation is reducing stress through relaxation. However, regular practice can have the benefit of shutting out the noise of everyday life and facilitating presence (also called mindfulness or being in the moment).

There are several examples of guided meditation practices available through YouTube, blogs, and other online resources.[18] Meditation apps, however, streamline the process of meditation and include steps to achieve new levels of meditation skills. There is no shortage of mindfulness and meditation apps that promise to help reduce anxiety, improve sleep quality, facilitate centeredness and focus, and provide other emotional and physical benefits. However, for a meditation and mindfulness app to be effective and user-friendly, there should be a significant number and variety of guided meditations available as the meditation practice progresses. Using the same series of meditations every day can become redundant, and a comprehensive, regularly updated content library can enhance the experience.[19] A well-designed meditation app is important; however, if the app design does not align with the user's self-care practice, it will not become a part of a regular meditation routine. A free trial for an app is important in a user's decision about which app is a good fit. Finally, meditation should be accessible to all users and in all locations, including on smartphones, smart watches, smart speakers, and web browsers. Available on devices, such as smart speakers, it allows users to meditate without picking up a phone.

Headspace20 (for meditation beginners) and Calm21 (for people who struggle to relax or sleep) are two examples of meditation apps. The opening screen on the *Head-space* app presents the "Today" view, which features that day's meditation, followed by the next meditation in any course (such as the basic introduction to medication), a daily wake-up video, and some guided breathing. *Headspace* offers options for sleep hygiene, including the Sleep tab, which has sleep meditations, Sleepcasts (sleep stories from people with soothing voices), sleep music, and an all-night relaxing sleep radio. *Headspace* offers a Move tab that includes several physical practices, including Feel Good Yoga and Mindful Cardio sessions, whereas the Focus tab has sessions and music to facilitate better work practices. *Headspace* takes a unique approach to beginners, including onboarding and three basic programs, which build on each other for consistency. Once onboarded, the structured courses allow the app user to move forward with the areas and techniques that are of most interest to them. *Headspace* offers one free basic course and requires a monthly fee for regular users.[20]

Calm, a favorite among meditation apps, makes meditation a part of daily life and an important self-care practice. On opening the app, the user is presented with suggested meditations, including The Daily Calm, which is a daily meditation. On opening the app again later in the day, the user receives a suggested sleep story. Sleep meditations feature smooth-voiced celebrities and meditation instructors telling stories that lull the listener to sleep. Some of the stories are traditional and intended to soothe, whereas others are deliberately boring. The app also includes other mindfulness and meditation features on the Meditate, Music, and More tabs.[21]

Habit Tracking

All humans have habits and rituals that they follow. They are the building blocks that form a large portion of what we do because they are essential for survival and a sustainable lifestyle. Without relying on habits that often put us on autopilot, we would be emotionally and mentally exhausted by the time we finished showering and brushing our teeth. By knowing this, we can "program" aspects of our personal autopilot modes, and by intentionally choosing and developing habits, we can determine how our future self-will react automatically when we do not have the time to consider what we are doing. Developing these habits can be challenging and time-consuming, but a habit-tracking app can help by engaging the user in a form of self-monitoring.[22] The user needs to consistently track relevant data that aligns with desired outcomes for the habit-tracking app to work effectively and efficiently. Habit tracking may also provide additional strategies for managing stress, anxiety, and depression, which impact caregiver well-being and resiliency.[22]

A habit tracker provides ways for the user to visualize patterns of actions (behaviors) that the user wants to reinforce or possibly change. *Habitify*[23] has an easy-to-use interface and user-friendly processes. The user inputs into the program what he/she wants to track, sets a reminder for multiple times a day (if desired), and monitors performance. For example, if the user wanted to increase his/her overall activity and movement levels, he/she could set specific times to "get moving" with a reminder and monitor steps, types of movement, and other activities associated with this habit. Performance data helps the user understand behavior (performance) over time, knowing that if more data is available, it will be easier to uncover patterns and guide behavioral actions to develop realistic goals.[23]

Habitica,[24] another habit tracker, appeals to gamers. Through an avatar in a role-playing game format, over time, the user's real-life actions impact the life of their avatar. The user can level up to earn rewards and unlock special features. *Habitica* offers the user the opportunity to address worrisome habits with friends. This can be effective and rewarding given there are 4 million Habiticans to potentially interact with.[24] *Coach.me*[25] is a habit tracker app for those who are ready to commit to developing good habits. The user can work with personal coaches along with standard habit tracker functionality. There is also support from the *Coach.me* community.[25]

Wearable Technology and Lifestyle Apps

Wearable technology, commonly known as wearables, signifies devices that individuals wear to analyze, track, and transfer personal data. These are smart devices designed to track biometric data ranging from sleep patterns to heart rate. Adopting wearable technology and lifestyle apps can also offer a multitude of strategies and techniques to better understand the physical and emotional connection to burnout, anxiety, and depression.[26] By helping employees make those connections, clinical leaders can take an integrated approach to building HWE for greater clinician well-being and resiliency.

Individuals and organizations use wearables to accurately transmit essential exercise, biological, and medical information to a database.[27] Informatics specialists report that artificial intelligence, robots, smart sensors, big data, radar technologies, and digital wearables may be more effective in managing and preventing diseases. These wearables and lifestyle apps can estimate blood pressure, body temperature, heart rate, and respiration of the young as well as the elderly. They can indicate risks, such as declining health, worsening diseases, and other threatening situations, including changes in blood glucose, increased blood pressure, and respiratory irregularities.[27] More than 80% of consumers leaned positively toward monitoring their health, tracking their vital signs, and applying wearable devices.[27]

Wearable devices are primarily used in the health and fitness sectors. An advantage of the wearables is that they allow users to transfer health data to health care professionals in real time. However, the primary risk of using wearable technologies is the lack of regulations and supervision over how they collect and transfer the data.[27] Popular wearable products include smart watches, smart glasses, hearables, head-mounted displays, sports watches, fitness trackers, and temperature controllers.[27] Constantly reviewing feedback from smart watches or fitness trackers has become a part of everyday life for millions of people across the world. These watches innately foster healthier lifestyles with their ability to collect large amounts of data and summarize it on easy-to-read interfaces. For example, knowing how far you can run may motivate you to push yourself harder to win against your previous record. Tracking your existing sleep habits can lead you to shifts in sleep behavior that will help you sleep more soundly. In other words, fitness trackers and smartwatches are some of the best tools to promote the health and fitness journey.[27]

There are pros and cons to wearable technologies. Increasing employee productivity, employee satisfaction, and enabling organizations to track employee health are positive aspects of engaging with wearable technology. For example, by using wearables, organizations can track the health and fitness of staff members as part of their health programs. The data collected by these devices are often correlated with incentive programs to reduce health care costs.[27]

There are downsides to wearables, including their lack of ability to operate as a standalone device, requiring a corresponding application on a smartphone or a tablet. This can increase administrative costs for organizations that provide wearables to their employees. Because wearables are always connected to the Internet, cyberattacks can be a security risk as they may not always be rigorously encrypted to protect personal data. Despite the risks of wearable technology and lifestyle apps, they can be effective and efficient strategies to reduce burnout, compassion fatigue, and tension in the workplace. Having strategies to connect to others in the workplace can increase an individual's ability to feel greater engagement with work, thus reducing feelings of isolation and going it alone.

Workplace Exemplar

Using information technology can enhance a health care system's ability to mitigate burnout and increase employee resilience. Health care systems that implement burnout reduction strategies for nurses through wage increases, professional mobility, stress reduction, and opportunities for learning and leadership spend about one-third less per year on costs related to nurse turnover attributable to burnout than hospitals without such initiatives.[28]

One example of an employee well-being program comes from the University of Virginia (UVA) Health.[28] At UVA Health, a program called *Wisdom & Wellbeing* helps health care staff reduce burnout by addressing sources of "stress injuries." Specifically, occupational trauma that triggers debilitating distress, anxiety, substance abuse, and even post-traumatic stress syndrome (PTSD) has been attributed to work strain (stress injuries) and can be addressed by building peer support, education, and on-unit consulting.[28] Stress injuries have enormous human and fiscal costs, including turnover, absenteeism, and reduced work productivity. Despite the great attention paid to these concerns during the pandemic, Muir and colleagues[28] noted that few hospitals routinely and intentionally measure burnout and its link to attrition. Valid and reliable measurements of burnout, such as the Maslach Burnout Inventory, are critical to developing a deeper understanding of the problem because exit surveys may lack consistency across units and result in ambiguous responses about leaving for "personal reasons" or because "the hours don't work for me."

Using results from measuring burnout, UVA was able to tailor their approach to address this critical concern, particularly related to reimbursement. To counteract stress and burnout, UVA Health offered a $3000 bonus to full-time nurses and a $1500 to part-time nurses to improve hiring and retention during the summer of 2021 and made plans to distribute more than $30 million in salary adjustments among its staff, including its nurses, starting in early 2022.[28]

Mentoring Programs

Face-to-face interaction between mentor and mentee in a physical space is typically regarded as the gold standard for professional coaching in the workplace by traditional mentoring programs. The pandemic provided opportunities to reimagine mentoring approaches, such as communicating in a digital or virtual environment (emailing, texting, chatting via messenger programs or social media, video conferencing) between mentors and mentees. Digital natives (people born between 1980 and 2010) are particularly comfortable in virtual and online environments, and intergenerational mentoring provides a meaningful way to keep the intellectual capital of baby boomers in an organization and aligns with the social needs of younger nurses.[29]

An excellent example of electronic monitoring is evident in the Catholic Health System, which, in 2014, launched a virtual care model to leverage nursing expertise.[30] This exemplar model uses a technology platform and a two-way camera to connect the expert nurse with patients and the care team. This mentoring program allows the nurse to remotely monitor up to 12 patients simultaneously and support the bedside nurse in aspects of care that do not require physical interventions.[30] The advantages of this model allow the remote nurse to appear on a monitor in the patient's room and respond to patient questions or virtually join and consult with the provider during clinical rounds. Serving in this virtual nursing role could delay the retirement of baby boomer nurses by creating an environment that capitalizes on the skills of the expert nurses while reducing the physical demands of the bedside. This exemplar, called the emeritus nurse (E-RN) model, is supportive of the workforce while possibly delaying the retirements of experienced nurses.[30] The intention is for retired or ready-to-retire RNs to offer respite for nurses during the workday. Specifically, the E-RN works 4-hour shifts in a role underpinned by their nursing knowledge while de-emphasizing their physical requirements. E-RNs typically focus on a variety of much-needed skills, including patient flow, the patient experience, mentoring, and quality improvement initiatives. The E-RN program has been effective, with one hospital that incorporated E-RNs demonstrating reduced turnover and $200,000 in cost savings in the first year.[30]

SUMMARY

Professional burnout is a significant occupational hazard, leading to lower job commitment, poor patient outcomes, reduced performance, lower job satisfaction, and frequent absenteeism. Advancing evidence-based, multidisciplinary solutions to improve patient care by caring for the caregiver is a cornerstone to increasing resiliency, well-being, empathy, and gratitude. Developing resilience in health care includes a wide array of technological methods to facilitate well-being. Digital journaling, mood tracking, meditation apps, habit tracking, lifestyle apps, and wearable technology facilitate healthy ways to deal with stress and compassion fatigue. Technology-enhanced mentorship support models also hold promise in bolstering nurse resilience and retention.

CLINICS CARE POINTS

- Resilience and a focus on worker well-being are protective factors against adversity and contribute to effective adaption to the burden of burnout.
- Nursing units that intentionally create a healthy work environment demonstrate better overall health of the work environment, better nurse staffing and retention, less moral distress, and lower rates of workplace violence.
- Through regularly assessing burnout and well-being, health care administrators can adjust salaries and bonus cycles, create well-being programs, and expand professional development practices to anticipate and prevent nurse attrition.
- Lifestyle apps and wearables, such as digital journaling, mood tracking, meditation apps, and habit tracking are technological strategies that can integrate healthy ways to deal with stress, compassion fatigue, and daily self-care practices.
- Employee well-being programs help health care staff overcome burnout by dealing with sources of "stress injuries," defined as occupational trauma that contributes to work strain by building peer support, education, and on-unit consulting.

DISCLOSURE

The author has nothing to disclose.

REFERENCES

1. Helliwell J, Layard R, Sachs J, et al. World Happiness Report 2019. Available at: https://www.hbs.edu/ris/Publication%20Files/WHR19_AW_a5c873ef-cc77-40df-aec0-c78ad3680b35.pdf. Accessed February 20, 2022.

2. Goh J, Pfeffer J, Zenios S. Exposure to Harmful Workplace Practices Could Account for Inequality in Life Spans Across Different Demographic Groups. Health Aff (Millwood) 2015;34(10):1761–8.

3. National Academies of Sciences, Engineering, and Medicine; National Academy of Medicine; Committee on the Future of Nursing 2020–2030. In: Flaubert JL, Le Menestrel S, Williams DR, et al, editors. The future of nursing 2020-2030: charting a path to achieve health equity. Washington, DC: National Academies Press (US); 2021.

4. Reith TP. Burnout in United States healthcare professionals: a narrative review. Cureus 2018;10(12):e3681.

5. How to Quit Your Job in the Great Post-Pandemic Resignation Boom. Bloomberg Business Week. 2021. Available at: https://www.bloomberg.com/news/articles/2021-05-10/quit-your-job-how-to-resign-after-covid-pandemic. Accessed February 19, 2022.

6. Professor who predicted "The Great Resignation' shares the 3 trends that will dominate work in 2022. 2022. Available at: https://www.cnbc.com/2022/01/14/the-great-resignation-expert-shares-the-biggest-work-trends-of-2022.html. Accessed February 1, 2022.

7. Job Openings and Labor Turnover Survey (JOLTS). 2021. Available at: https://www.bls.gov/jlt/. Accessed February 1, 2022.

8. Dyrbye LN, Meyers D, Ripp J, et al. A pragmatic approach for organizations to measure health care professional well-being. NAM perspectives. Washington, DC: National Academy of Medicine; 2018. https://doi.org/10.31478/201810b. Available at:.

9. American Association of Critical Care Nurses. Healthy work environments. Available at: https://www.aacn.org/nursing-excellence/healthy-work-environments. Accessed February 2, 2022.

10. Perlo J, Balik B, Swensen S, et al. IHI framework for improving joy in work. IHI white paper. Cambridge, Massachusetts: Institute for Healthcare Improvement; 2017. Available at ihi.org.

11. Ohren N, Adams K, Hudson B. The 30-day digital journaling challenge a report for helping professionals. Cent J Ther 2015;10:13.

12. Therapeutic Journaling: Susan Borkin's "The Healing Power of Writing". 2015. Available at: https://www.mindingtherapy.com/therapeutic-journaling/. Accessed February 2, 2022.

13. The 8 best journal apps of 2021. Available at: https://zapier.com/blog/best-journaling-apps/. Accessed February 2, 2022.

14. Day One. Your journal for Life. Available at: https://dayoneapp.com/. Accessed February 2, 2022.

15. Memento. capture your Life. Available at: https://momentoapp.com/. Accessed February 2, 2022.

16. Daylio. Self-care bullet journal with goals mood diary & happiness tracker. Available at: https://daylio.net/. Accessed February 2, 2022.

17. Journaling to reduce COVID-19 stress. Michigan State University Extension. 2020. Available at: https://www.canr.msu.edu/news/journaling_to_reduce_stress. Accessed February 2, 2022.

18. Best Meditation Apps Recharge and relax, Improve focus, and more. 2021. Available at: https://www.verywellmind.com/best-meditation-apps-4767322. Accessed February 2, 2022.

19. The 5 best meditation apps in 2021. Available at: https://zapier.com/blog/best-meditation-app/. Accessed February 2, 2022.

20. Headspace. Meditation and mindfulness for any mind, any mood, any goal. Available at: https://www.headspace.com/. Accessed February 2, 2022.

21. Find your Calm. Available at: https://www.calm.com/. Accessed February 2, 2022.

22. Best habit tracker apps in 2021 to keep your mental health right. 2020. Available at: https://www.calmsage.com/best-habit-tracker-apps/#:~:text=Best%20Habit %20Tracker%20Apps%3A%201%20Habitify.%20All%20the,habits.%20.%204% 20Beeminder.%20.%205%20Strides.%20. Accessed February 2, 2022.

23. Build Golden Habits, Unlock your Potential. Available at: https://www.habitify.me/. Accessed February 2, 2022.

24. Motivate Yourself to Achieve Your Goals. Available at: https://habitica.com/static/ home. Accessed February 2, 2022.

25. Coach.me. Available at: https://www.coach.me/habit-tracker. Accessed February 2, 2022.

26. The top health wearables for A healthy lifestyle. Available at: https:// medicalfuturist.com/top-health-wearables/. Accessed February 2, 2022.

27. Wearable Technology: Wearable Devices for Health Monitoring purpose. 2021. Available at: https://digitalhealth.folio3.com/blog/wearable-device-for-health-monitoring/. Accessed February 2, 2022.

28. Muir JK, Wanchek T, Lobo J, et al. Evaluating the costs of nurse burnout-attributed turnover: A markov modeling approach. J Patient Saf 2021. https:// doi.org/10.1097/PTS.0000000000000920.

29. Gaffney T. Retaining nurses to mitigate shortages. Am Nurse 2022;17(1):14–25. Available at: https://www.myamericannurse.com/wp-content/uploads/2022/01/ an1-Beyond-Retention-1213.pdf.

30. Rehired. Emeritus nurses bring knowledge and experience to younger workforce. 2020. Available at: https://campaignforaction.org/rehired-emeritus-nurses-bring-knowledge-and-experience-to-younger-workforce/. Accessed February 2, 2022.

Addressing Challenges to the Development, Delivery, and Evaluation of Continuing Education for Nurses

Elisa C. Jang, DNP, MS, RN, CNS, EBP-C

KEYWORDS

- Clinical nurse specialist • Continuing nursing education
- Educational needs assessment • Educational technology • Gamification
- Nursing staff • Simulation training • Staff development • competency assessment

KEY POINTS

- The development of continuing education starts with performing a thorough learning needs assessment.
- Delivery of continuing education needs to be implemented using a multimodal approach which accommodates various learning preferences and incorporates adult learning principles.
- Simulation training and gamification are emerging trends in continuing education that can provide an interactive and engaging experience for the learner.
- Fellowship programs, interprofessional education, simulation, and nurse-led research programs provide comprehensive strategies to fill practice gaps and deliver continuing education.
- Collaboration between nurse educators, clinical nurse specialists, and clinical nurse leaders can enhance the development, delivery, and evaluation of continuing education.

Registered nurses are accountable for demonstrating professional competency through the ongoing completion of continuing education. According to the American Nurses Association, the employer shares responsibility with the nurse for staying up to date with current nursing knowledge and is accountable for providing an environment favorable to competent practice.[1] Moreover, patients want assurance that nurses are competent in current nursing knowledge, skills, and abilities (KSAs) so they can provide the care that is needed. However, in the current dynamic health care environment, employers and professional nurses face challenges in ensuring

Leadership Institute, Center for Nursing Excellence & Innovation, UCSF Health 2001 The Embarcadero, suite 1100, San Francisco, CA 94143
E-mail address: elisa.jang@ucsf.edu

Nurs Clin N Am 57 (2022) 513–523
https://doi.org/10.1016/j.cnur.2022.06.003
0029-6465/22/© 2022 Elsevier Inc. All rights reserved.

nurses can complete the required continuing education necessary to meet expectations set by governmental agencies that regulate nursing practice.

The guarantee of competence is a responsibility shared by individual nurses, professional organizations, credentialing and certification bodies, regulatory agencies, employers, and other key stakeholders.[1] Professional development plays a crucial role in sustaining and verifying the competence of a registered nurse. The need to provide ongoing education utilizing technology and a creative approach is more important than ever to keep a multi-generational, multicultural nursing workforce engaged in continuous learning.

BACKGROUND

Nurses across all clinical settings face the task of staying abreast of the latest evidence and clinical practice guidelines, regulatory mandates, clinical practice changes, equipment updates, and other workplace requirements.[2] Both scientific and technological progress, along with increased patient care demands and needs, pose challenges for nurses to maintain their skills and motivation to engage in the continuous education required to provide safe care to patients.[3] Many barriers can pose a risk to providing continuing education, such as lack of time, burnout, limited access to resources, lack of flexibility in educational approaches, financial constraints, and staffing issues.[3,4] Employers do not want nurses to spend time away from the bedside to complete training, and nurses do not want to spend time in a classroom listening passively to a didactic lecture. This conundrum demands that nursing professional development (NPD) practitioners develop, deliver, and evaluate engaging, efficient, and effective continuing education opportunities to keep up with the ever-changing health care environment where quality and safe patient care must be maintained. How do institution-based nurse educators ensure participation, completion, and comprehensive assessments of continuing education opportunities?

GOALS IN CONTINUING EDUCATION

The dynamic nature of health care combined with the impact of the pandemic calls for a change in continuous professional education and how it is delivered. Strategies for continuing education need to include integrated learning and interactive, engaging teaching strategies.[4] The application of evidence-based theoretic learning frameworks will help keep NPD practitioners grounded in standards of practice and standards of care. By utilizing a conceptual framework, NPD practitioners can design and develop continuing education in an environment that supports a culture of professional development and lifelong learning. The Nursing Professional Development Practice model (**Fig. 1**) describes the teaching and learning process as an input-throughput-output system.[5] The inputs include both the NPD practitioners and the learners. The throughputs represent the various kinds of learning activities that NPD practitioners can offer and nurses can engage in. The outputs are elements of professional role competence and growth.

The environment in which the learning takes place can vary depending on what is available within each organization. The goal of the NPD practitioners is to capture the dynamic nature of lifelong learning and create a positive and engaging learning environment in which nurses can participate in continuing professional development. The partnership between individual nurses and NPD practitioners is integral in making this a successful experience with the goals of gaining KSAs, advancing clinical practice, and improving patient outcomes.

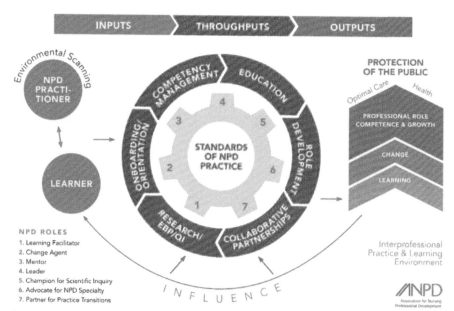

Fig. 1. Nursing professional development practice model. EBP, evidence-based practice; QI, quality improvement. © 2016 ANPDP. Used with permission.

DESIGN AND DEVELOPMENT OF CONTINUING EDUCATION
Learning Needs Assessment

The first step in designing and developing a continuing education program is to perform a learning needs assessment of practice gaps. Findings from the learning needs assessment will reveal the topics that need to be covered and which competencies need to be verified through continuing education. NPD practitioners can approach a learning needs assessment through direct observation of clinical practice at the microsystem level, staff surveys of personally identified learning needs, evaluation of areas needing improvement in quality benchmark outcomes, and analysis of trends in organization-specific risk management systems.

The Donna Wright Competency Assessment model[6] is a framework that can be used to identify practice gaps and select and verify competencies in continuing professional education. This model is composed of three distinguishing elements of success: ownership, empowerment, and accountability (**Fig. 2**). Ownership refers to nurses' owning their practice and, therefore, owning their own competencies. Empowerment refers to putting each employee at the center of the verification process and empowering them to bring the evidence of their own competency forward. Accountability refers to the culture where leaders provide the organizational mission while supporting the employee's ability to be accountable to do the best work possible. According to the Donna Wright Competency model, competency assessment is a fluid, ongoing process that helps identify and evaluate the skills that are necessary to carry out a job in its current and future state as the job evolves.[7] Identification of potential competencies is accomplished by asking four basic questions:

1. What are the NEW procedures, policies, equipment, initiatives, and so forth that affect this job class?
2. What are the CHANGES in procedures, policies, equipment, initiatives, and so forth that affect this job class?

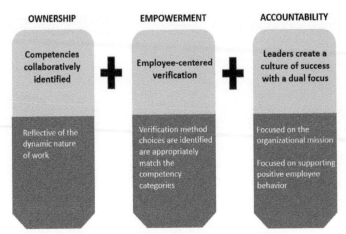

Fig. 2. Donna Wright competency model (Wright, 2021). Used with permission. © 2005, Donna Wright/Creative Health Care Management, Inc. www.chcm.com.

3. What are the HIGH-RISK aspects of this job? (High risk is anything that would cause harm, death, or legal action to an individual or an organization.)
4. What are the PROBLEMATIC aspects of this job? (These can be identified through quality monitoring, incident reports, patient surveys, staff surveys, and any other form of formal or informal evaluation.)[8]

This approach keeps the practice gaps at the forefront, including assessing all domains of skill (technical, critical thinking, and interpersonal). The model facilitates the process for NPD practitioners to select which competencies are prioritized by providing an opportunity for nurses, NPD practitioners, and nursing unit leaders to participate in the process.

Another unique feature of the Donna Wright competency model is the approach to how competencies are verified. Traditionally, return demonstration has been the hallmark of how NPD practitioners can be assured that nurses are competent in a particular skill. This approach can be problematic due to current challenges with staffing shortages and a need to keep nurses at the point of care instead of pulling them from their duties to demonstrate competency in a skills laboratory. The Donna Wright model offers 11 different categories of competency verification methods (**Table 1**). Each method assesses and measures a specific domain of skill. By providing several options to measure a competency, NPD practitioners contribute to building a culture of autonomy and empowerment. This approach builds on existing adult learning principles, which typically underpin successful competency-based learning, into a competency-based program and creates employee and leadership buy-in.[9]

Approaches to the Delivery of Continuing Education

Once the learning needs assessment has been completed, continuing education opportunities can be created to fill gaps in practice. Delivery of education in a traditional didactic lecture format in a classroom is no longer sufficient to meet the needs of the health care workforce. Continuing education needs to be delivered in multimodal formats, such as clinical update documents, competency assessments, e-learning modules, webinars, workshops, conferences, specialty certifications, and simulation training.[3] For example, a self-directed learning module coupled with coaching support in the clinical areas can help to facilitate and sustain practice improvement.[5]

Table 1
Donna Wright model verification methods[8]

Methods of Verification	Definitions
Tests	Written test, quizzes, oral exams, surveys, worksheets, calculation tests, crossword puzzles, and word games
Return demonstration	An individual demonstrates a set of skills for a skilled observer.
Evidence of daily work	Skills demonstrated in the work setting
Case studies	Describes a situation and asks individuals to explain their responses or choices
Exemplars	A story you tell or write yourself that describes a situation and rationale about choices you made.
Peer review/feedback	Process of assessing, monitoring, and making judgments about the quality of practice and care provided by a peer
Self-assessment	Assessing one's values, beliefs, opinions, and attitudes
Discussion/reflection groups	Group of individuals share thoughts and strategies on an issue and discuss merits of each aspect
Presentations	Share information gained from experience or through an educational event
Mock events/surveys	Simulations of real-life situations carried out in a work setting, skills laboratory/fair, or simulation center
Quality monitors	Checks compliance and document adherence to policies/procedures/protocols

Assessing competencies through verification methods, such as those suggested in the Donna Wright model, can also serve as a guide in the design and delivery of continuing education. Participants in continuing education events come with various learning needs and preferences; so, offering multiple formats should become the norm. In-person or virtual meetings, synchronous versus asynchronous formats, hybrid delivery, flipped classroom (an instructional strategy in which students complete readings at home and work on problem-solving during class time), and use of simulation and learning technologies need to be considered in relation to the audience, educational content, instructional delivery context, and availability of resources.

Fellowship programs

One method of offering continuing education is through a fellowship program. The concept of a fellowship program has been documented in the literature as an innovative strategy to narrow the gap of translating research into clinical practice.[10,11] A fellowship program can be used as part of a comprehensive strategic plan to support clinicians in the discovery and application of new evidence-based clinical practices to improve patient care, quality, and safety. Benefits of fellowship programs include support for evidence-based practice (EBP) principles, acquisition of up-to-date clinical knowledge and abilities, integration of the best evidence with clinical practice, and promotion of innovative thinking regarding practice that can improve patient outcomes.[10] A qualitative study on an EBP fellowship program revealed that fellows felt empowered, more confident and knowledgeable, and gained additional opportunities in their professional growth due to their participation in the program.[12] A fellowship program offers continuing education that motivates nurses to participate in lifelong learning with two dimensions: (1) intrinsic (personal growth) and (2) extrinsic (external forces, such as improving patient care, clinical advancement, or professional goals). Fellowship programs as a form of continuing education promote cooperative learning in which students can engage in social learning and develop professionally as part of a group with other learners.

Nurse-led research programs

In addition, nurse-led research is increasingly recognized as a critical pathway to practical and efficient ways of reducing hospital errors, decreasing unnecessary costs, and improving patient outcomes.[13] A clinical research fellowship program in Melbourne, Australia used a multidisciplinary approach, including 15 participants representing various departments within the hospital in their EBP and research program.[14] More than half of the EBP projects resulted in finding evidence to support practice changes, whereas the remainder of the EBP projects generated research questions that were answered when fellowship participants engaged in primary research activities. This study also highlights the important role of fellowship programs as a means for health care organizations to adopt a culture of EBP and improve clinical outcomes by engaging employees through an interactive approach to continuing education.

Interprofessional education and practice

Several studies have also shown that an interprofessional educational approach affects both knowledge and confidence.[15–17] Interdisciplinary team training has been effective not only in increasing knowledge and confidence but also in improving clinical practice in fall prevention and pain management.[17,18] The British Department of Health recommends that professionals in the health and social services adopt an evidence-based interdisciplinary collaborative approach so that patients can receive appropriate care.[19] Interprofessional education has also been endorsed by the Institute of Healthcare Improvement as an important transition in health care that will further the "triple aim" by encouraging teamwork among health care professionals.[15] With the updated goals for the quadruple aim, interprofessional partnerships gained through participating in education together has the potential to positively affect workplace well-being and job satisfaction.[20]

The development and design of interprofessional education is not as simple as bringing a group of people together from different health care disciplines. A quasi-experimental study revealed that barriers to the delivery of interprofessional education do exist and need to be taken into consideration in the design of learning experiences.[18] Some of the barriers to delivering interprofessional education that were encountered included lack of consistent and equal access to technology among health care professionals; providing education through online modules only; lack of protected time and organizational support; and scheduling educational opportunities that do not accommodate the work schedules of all involved individuals.

Simulation

Simulation-based training strategies promote a safe, positive learning environment while providing a structured, engaging, and effective delivery methodology.[21] Simulation allows for a broad range of technical skills and can also facilitate the learning of soft skills, including teamwork, communication, and collaboration. Simulation training does not always need to occur in a simulation center or skills laboratory. In situ simulation is a blended approach involving the use of either high- or low-fidelity patient simulators within an actual clinical environment.[21] Simulation training helps nurses understand the relevance of a specific focal topic and keeps the nurses closer to the point of care by providing continuing education in the area where they work.

Role of Technology in Continuing Education

Educational technology has become more affordable and accessible, and NPD practitioners need to stay abreast of the multitude of options that are available for continuing education. The use of learning management systems (LMSs) is one option, and some LMSs come with content already developed and ready for online module delivery, such as Cornerstone and Lippincott Learning. Mobile learning apps can also be utilized to promote active engagement in learning. While the possibilities for incorporating technology into continuing education are seemingly limitless, NPD practitioners must evaluate which options are the best fit for the content they need to deliver, the learners who will interact with the technology, and the organization (**Table 2**).

Gamification is an emerging trend in health care education that involves using game-based elements, such as point scoring, peer competition, teamwork, and score tables, in a nongame environment. Gamification can drive interactive learning and interest from the learner, in addition to increasing learners' motivation, problem-solving abilities, and knowledge retention.[22,23] Gamification is a more engaging way to

---

Table 2
Examples of educational technology

Educational Technology	Descriptions
Learning management system	Software application for administration, documentation, tracking, and delivery of educational courses
Interactive whiteboards/smartboards	Interactive touchscreen connected to a computer and projectors that can be manipulated with a finger or pen
Virtual reality or augmented reality	Used with specific apps to provide a 360-degree view. Virtual reality/augmented reality can evoke emotional reactions, increase empathy, and enhance learning.
Digital readers and tablets	Handheld devices that enable students to have greater interaction with the material covered through mixed media
Video conferencing	Can connect learners from different locations and allow students to participate in the same lesson at a convenient place for each learner
Cloud servers	Students are able to access all of the learning materials they need through a cloud-based system
Three-dimensional printing	Ability to create hands-on models that students can investigate and interact with
Artificial intelligence	Artificial intelligence is intelligence demonstrated by a machine. It can help with evaluating outcomes of learning and providing personalized feedback.
Mobile technology	Provides educational or interactive apps for students to engage in their own learning process
Podcasts	Can provide supplemental lessons in a meaningful way and encourages auditory learning
Quick response codes	Type of barcode that can contain links to learning materials

provide professional development than traditional didactic lecture. Students learn better when they are having fun.[24] The use of gaming in continuing education ties together the fun element of play with the content and concepts that nurses must learn. There are three basic elements involved in gamification: (1) game-based mechanics (rules, challenges, points, interactivity, and so forth.); (2) esthetics (visual appeal of the gamification environment, such as presentation design); and (3) game thinking (integrating elements of competition, cooperation, and exploration).[24] One example of an innovative gamification strategy for teaching is the use of an escape room. An escape room combines elements of simulation and gamification through an immersive learning environment. Nurses apply concepts learned from a class, an e-learning module, or a workshop to obtain clues to progress through the simulation.[25]

Collaborations in Nursing Professional Development Practice

It is important for NPD practitioners to create collaborative avenues that will help nurses in their professional development. NPD practitioners should create partnerships with clinical nurse specialists (CNSs) and clinical nurse leaders (CNLs) who can provide significant support in the design, delivery, and evaluation of continuing education. An analysis of the CNS and CNL roles is important to understanding how they can collaborate with nurse educators in the design, development, and implementation of continuing education. Nurse educators are master's-prepared nurses who have been trained in instructional design and adult learning principles to facilitate learning in the clinical setting and assess nursing clinical performance.[26] CNSs are advanced practice registered nurses who have graduate-level preparation and are trained in physiology, pharmacology, and physical assessment, in addition to their specific areas of specialty. They provide clinical expertise, support nurses who care for patients, and drive practice change throughout organizations.[27] CNLs are graduate-level advanced generalists who facilitate, coordinate, and oversee care within the microsystem and macrosystem of a healthcare organization.[28]

CNSs can start the process of continuing education development by performing a gap analysis through evaluation of the latest standards of practice and standards of care, examining quality improvement data, and gauging any upcoming organizational initiatives. They can work collaboratively with nurse educators and CNLs to conduct a literature review on any new clinical practice guidelines or updates within each of their respective units or departments. Once the learning needs assessment has been completed, all three roles can work together to develop a plan for the delivery of continuing education that meets both organization-wide and unit-based needs. Nurse educators can then develop lesson plans and courses by utilizing the various delivery and teaching methodologies that are available within their organization. Once the continuing education is delivered, CNLs can contribute to the evaluation of learning outcomes by assessing whether nurses are applying theory to practice and ensuring standardization of practices is sustained and meeting quality outcomes. The nurse educator, CNS, and CNL make a powerful trio in the design and delivery of continuing education that can elevate clinical practice, drive positive change, and improve clinical outcomes.

DISCUSSION

Staying up-to-date with continuing education requirements has become a challenging issue for nurses, NPDs, and employers in recent years due to staffing shortages, financial constraints brought on by the consequences of the pandemic and increasing health care costs, and constant change in health care. Quality outcomes, meeting benchmarks, and patient and employee satisfaction are all regular topics in leadership meetings that occur on a daily basis. Many of these challenges can be addressed by improving organizational systems, updating technology, and providing a strong organizational infrastructure that supports administrators, interdisciplinary clinicians, and nurses to provide safe patient care.

Organizational infrastructure and culture play a significant supporting role in the success of continuing education efforts. However, limitations on dedicated time for training and education for nurses during scheduled working hours can interfere with moving clinical practice changes and quality improvement efforts forward. An insufficient number of nurse educators and a lack of administrative support also impede practice. Health care systems can demonstrate their commitment to supporting continuing professional education for nurses by providing resources and funding for educational activities and technology. Nurse educators can provide invaluable guidance in the professional development process, and support from nursing management can reduce or eliminate barriers to implementation of change processes.

Continuing education serves as a pathway to improving practice and will continue to be a necessary and crucial part of professional nursing practice. NPD practitioners shoulder a large portion of the responsibility for the development, delivery, and evaluation of continuing education but should also seek opportunities for collaboration with CNSs and CNLs. Continuing education development can be accomplished through assessments of learning needs in both the microsystem and macrosystem. Finding creative and innovative approaches to teaching will help nurse educators meet clinical goals while evaluating whether the educational methods were successful in helping nurses meet the focal learning objectives. The use of technology, such as mobile apps, simulation training, and gamification, is becoming more accessible and easier to implement. NPD practitioners must stay current with the latest learning and health care technologies and communicate to health care leaders the importance of taking advantage of these resources within their organization.

SUMMARY

Continuing education provides a pathway for professional nurses to stay-up-to date with their clinical KSAs. A very specific set of skills and processes is needed by NPD practitioners to execute successful educational programs. The process starts with performing a gap analysis, which helps focus and drive the development of continuing education topics. An understanding of adult learning principles, learning preferences, and various teaching and learning strategies is crucial in the design and delivery of professional learning opportunities. Fellowship programs, simulation training, and gamification present innovative possibilities to address current barriers to empowering nurses to own their competency and accountability for professional development. Readily available options in educational technology can help NPD practitioners find a strategy that supports practice advancement and quality, safe patient care through continuing education.

Continuing education supports a lifelong learning paradigm that nursing as a profession has a responsibility to promote. Continuing education will continue to play a crucial role in sustaining nurses' competence in an ever changing and complex health care environment. Florence Nightingale knew the importance of continuing education, as she is quoted to say, "Let us never consider ourselves finished nurses. We must be learning all of our lives."[29] Nurses are uniquely positioned at all levels of practice to ask the burning clinical questions, engage in the advancement of nursing practice through continuing education, and achieve the best possible clinical outcomes.

CLINICS CARE POINTS

- Continuing education supports nursing professional development and lifelong learning through continual quality improvement in nursing and advancement in clinical practice.
- Continuing education is a responsibility shared by professional nurses, employers, and nursing professional development practitioners.
- Frameworks and models such as the Nursing Professional Development Practice model and the Donna Wright Competency model can facilitate the design, delivery, and evaluation of continuing education.
- Educational technologies are readily available to facilitate delivery of multimodal, engaging, and interactive continuing education opportunities for busy nurses.
- Collaboration between three clinical roles in health care (nurse educators, clinical nurse specialists, and clinical nurse leaders) is key to providing flexible, engaging continuing education opportunities and evaluating learning outcomes.

DISCLOSURE

The author has nothing to disclose.

REFERENCES

1. Nurses Association American. Position statement on professional role competence. In: American nurses association. 2014. Available at: https://nursingworld.org/practice-policy/nursing-excellence/official-position-statement/id/professional-role-competence/. Accessed December 27, 2021.
2. Bindon SL. Professional development strategies to enhance nurses' knowledge and maintain safe practice. Assoc Perioper Registered Nurses J 2017;106(2): 99–110.
3. Vazquez-Calatayud M, Errasti-Ibarrondo B, Choperena A. Nurses' continuing professional development: A systematic literature review. Nurse Education Pract 2021;50:1–9.
4. Rheingans J. The nursing professional development practice model. J Nurses Prof Development 2016;32(5):278–81.
5. Duff B, Gardner G, Osborne S. An integrated educational model for continuing nurse education. Nurse Educ Today 2014;34(1):104–11.
6. Wright D. The goals of competency assessment. In: The ultimate guide to competency assessment in healthcare. Minneapolis (MN): Creative Health Care Management; 2021. p. xiii, 2.
7. Wright D. Elements of competency assessment. In: The ultimate guide to competency assessment in healthcare. Minneapolis (MN); 2021. p. 16.
8. Wright D. Ongoing competencies assessment: Ownership. In: The ultimate guide to competency assessment in healthcare. Minneapolis (MN); 2021. p. 30-31.
9. Wright D. Verification methods. In: The ultimate guide to competency assessment in healthcare. Minneapolis (MN); 2021. p. 63-136.
10. Selig PM, Estes TS, Nease B. Developing an evidence-based practice fellowship program. Newborn Infant Nurs Rev 2009;9(2):99–101.
11. Gawlinski A, Becker E. Infusing research into practice: A staff nurse evidence-based practice fellowship program. J Nurses Staff Dev 2012;28(2):69–73.

12. Christenbery T, Williamson A, Sandlin V, et al. Immersion in evidence-based practice fellowship program: A transforming experience for staff nurses. J Nurses Prof Development 2016;32(1):15–20.
13. Curtis K, Fry M, Shaban RZ, et al. Translating research findings to clinical nursing practice. J Clin Nurs 2016;26:862–72.
14. Milne DJ, Krishnasamy M, Johnston L, et al. Promoting evidence-based care through a clinical research fellowship programme. J Clin Nurs 2017;16(9): 1629–39.
15. Aronoff N, Stellrecht E, Lyons AG, et al. Teaching evidence-based practice principles to prepare health professions students for an interprofessional learning experience. J Med Libr Assoc JMLA. 2017;105(4):376–84.
16. Bennet S, Hoffmann T, Arkins M. A multi-professional evidence-based practice course improved allied health students' confidence and knowledge. J Eval Clin Pract 2011;17(4):635–9.
17. McKenzie G, Lasater K, Delander GE, et al. Falls prevention education: Interprofessional training to enhance collaborative practice. Gerontol Geriatr Educ 2017; 38(2):232–43.
18. Patel B, Hacker E, Murks CM, et al. Interdisciplinary pain education: Moving from discipline-specific to collaborative practice. Clin J Oncol Nurs 2016;20(6): 636–43.
19. Ndoro S. Effective multidisciplinary working: the key to high-quality care. Br J Nurs 2014;23(13):724–7.
20. Melnyk BM, Gallagher-Ford L, Zellefrow C, et al. Outcomes from the first Helene Fuld Health Trust National Institute for Evidence-Based Practice in Nursing and Healthcare invitational expert forum. Worldviews Evidence-Based Nurs 2018; 15(1):5–15.
21. Rosen MA, Hunt EA, Pronovost PJ, et al. In situ simulation in continuing education for the health care professions: A systematic review. J Contin Educ Health Prof 2012;32(4):243–54.
22. Subhash S, Cudney EA. Gamified learning in higher education: A systematic review of the literature. Comput Hum Behav 2018;87:192–206.
23. Marti-Parreno J, Mendez-Ibanez E, Alonso-Arroyo A. The use of gamification in education: a bibliographic and text mining analysis. J Computer Assisted Learn 2016;32:663–76.
24. Woolwine S, Romp CR, Jackson B. Game on: evaluating the impact of gamification in nursing orientation on motivation and knowledge retention. J Nurses Prof Development 2019;35(5):255–60.
25. Brown N, Darby W, Coronel H. An escape room as a simulation technology strategy. Clin Simulation Nurs 2019;30:1.
26. National League for Nursing. Nurse educator core competencies. 2021. Available at. http://www.nln.org/professional-development-programs/competencies-for-nursing-education/nurse-educator-core-competency/. Accessed January 9, 2022.
27. National Association of Clinical Nurse Specialists. What is a clinical nurse specialist?. 2021. Available at. https://nacns.org/about-us/what-is-a-cns/. Accessed January 9, 2022.
28. Clinical Nurse Leader Association. What is a CNL?. 2021. Available at. https://cnlassociation.org/what-is-a-cnl/. Accessed January 9, 2022.
29. Wilson C. The role of nursing professional development in the future of nursing. J Nurses Prof Development 2015;31(1):56–7.

The Power of Presence in Virtual Teaching and Practice Environments

Elizabeth Anne Crooks, DNP, RN, CNE*, Nancy P. Wingo, PhD, MA

KEYWORDS

- Educational technology • Family presence • Community of inquiry • Telemedicine
- Telepresence • Visitors to patients

KEY POINTS

- Family and nurse presence is essential to patient-centered care and can be facilitated with communication technology.
- Telepresence is the ability to provide human presence by using video chat when the ability to be physically present is not possible.
- The ethical, technical, and logistical issues that arise when using telepresence can be addressed by guidelines and processes that support using communication technology at the bedside.
- The Community of Inquiry model provides a framework for understanding how human presence is experienced in online learning encounters.
- Common challenges with virtual nursing instruction can be resolved with thoughtful instructional design that supports the user and fosters communication and collaboration.

INTRODUCTION

As COVID-19 spread across the globe, half of the world's population was locked down by the end of March 2020.[1] The impact of this unprecedented restriction in human movement could be observed on the ground and from outer space. People remained at home leaving public spaces empty, highways untraveled, and airplanes on the ground. As a result, the skies cleared and water became cleaner.[2] Human presence: it is a phenomenon felt by both humankind and Mother Nature.

The lack of human presence was also felt acutely within healthcare systems and nursing education. Hospitals and clinics closed their doors to everyone but the health team and the patient. Nursing schools suspended in-person classes and required educators and students to rapidly adopt virtual teaching and learning strategies. The

School of Nursing, University of Alabama at Birmingham, 1701 University Boulevard, Birmingham, AL 35294, USA
* Corresponding author.
E-mail address: eacrooks@uab.edu

Nurs Clin N Am 57 (2022) 525–538
https://doi.org/10.1016/j.cnur.2022.07.002
0029-6465/22/© 2022 Elsevier Inc. All rights reserved.

challenges that the COVID-19 pandemic posed to the effective use of presence in clinical settings and the classroom were unprecedented; however, the technological strategies used to address them speak to nursing's ingenuity and resilience.

PRESENCE IN CLINICAL NURSING PRACTICE

The most common sources of human presence for hospitalized patients are the patient's family and support persons, health team and hospital staff members, and nursing staff. During care coordination, nurses facilitate these types of presence to promote patient well-being. This discussion focuses on the impact COVID-19 had on family and support person presence and nurse presence for hospitalized adult patients.

Family/Support Person Presence

The benefits of having the patient's family member or support person present during times of acute and critical illness have been well described and are summarized in **Table 1**. As evidence for these benefits grew, the American Association of Critical Care Nurses supported the patient's unrestricted access to family members in acute and critical care settings and encouraged hospitals to liberalize visitation.[3] Recently, the ability for family members and support persons to remain physically present with their loved one, even during invasive procedures or cardiopulmonary resuscitation, has become more commonplace.

Nurses now have an ethical mandate to foster family and support-person's presence when a patient is isolated due to quarantine or hospitalization.[4] Family and support persons are no longer thought of as visitors whose presence is optional but rather as care partners whose presence is integral to providing patient-centered care.[5] In addition, The Nursing Intervention Classification (NIC) system addresses this practice and identifies "family presence facilitation" as a nursing intervention for use in support of such individuals.[6]

Unfortunately, the COVID-19 pandemic negatively impacted this practice. Based on guidance from the Center for Disease Control and Centers for Medicare and Medicaid, hospitals restricted family and support-person visits early in the pandemic to limit community spread.[11,12] As a result, patients and their families found themselves without the ability to be physically present for one another during a time when they faced significant health challenges like delivery of or hospitalization of a child, the need to undergo an urgent surgical procedure, serious illness, and for some, impending death.

The Shift to Family Telepresence

Telepresence via video chat has been proposed as a means of combatting social isolation and loneliness in older adults during times of restricted social activities due to the pandemic.[13] As the COVID-19 pandemic forced hospitals to shut their doors to visitors, nurses pivoted to digital technology and video communication platforms to create a space where patients and their family or support persons could engage remotely with one another and health team members. Cell phones are ubiquitous in the United States, and much of the public already has experience using smartphone video chat platforms. Nurses leveraged this technology to allow patients to communicate remotely with their loved ones when the physical presence of a loved one was not possible. In addition to cell phones, nurses also used web-based technologies to provide video chat or video conferencing. These technologies included handheld devices, such as iPads, and telehealth devices, mounted on carts for portability.

Table 1
Benefits of family/support person presence in adult acute and critical care settings

Physical Benefits[3,7]	Psychosocial Benefits[7–9]	Health System Benefits[8,10]
Fewer cardiovascular adverse events Decreased delirium	Reduced anxiety Improved cognition Improved patient communication Enhanced patient and family satisfaction	Improved patient safety Decreased intensive care unit length of stay Increased staff satisfaction

Patients with sufficient cognitive function and dexterity to use their own cell phone can generally manage their family's telepresence with minimal assistance. However, it is not unusual for patients to require help. This assistance often takes the form of (1) assisting the patient to use their own device; (2) assisting with the use a device on loan; (3) selecting and using a video chat application; (4) coordinating calls to family and support persons; and (5) coaching family and support persons on how to use video chat as a way of being present for their loved one.

The Nature of Telepresence

Telepresence has been defined in the computer science field as "the ability to interact (often via computer mediation) with a physically real, remote environment experienced from the first-person point of view."[14] Simply put, a person who is experiencing telepresence has the feeling they are present with those who are in a remote location. The concept of telepresence in nursing science is still being explored. Recently, Groom and colleagues[15] used dimensional analysis to examine the concept of telepresence in the clinical literature to gain insights into what makes a telehealth visit engaging and effective. Based on their findings, they proposed this definition for telepresence: "Telepresence is the patient's, caregiver's, and clinician's experienced realism during a telehealth encounter that is created through connection and collaboration built on trust, support, and the clinician's skill at acting as the technology mediator when the third actor (technology) influences the patient or caregiver or clinician interaction."[15] Although the context for this definition is a telehealth encounter rather than personal communication, it highlights how facilitating family telepresence is a collaborative effort between nurse, patient, and family that hinges on the nurse's ability to skillfully use video chat technology to provide a shared reality.

Telepresence has limitations. Sharing physical space provides the opportunity for participants to touch one another and more clearly communicate using non-verbal cues. This advantage is lost in remote encounters where two-dimensional images on audio/visual screens may make it difficult to discern body language and intended tone. The physical and verbal cues used to facilitate fluid conversation are also difficult to discern when using video chat platforms, and this can lead to crosstalk and difficulty managing conversations among multiple people. When emotions run high, it can be difficult for parties to be fully heard and understood.

Visual distractions from activity in the background can be confusing to video chat users. Some video chat platforms allow the user to blur the background so that the focus is on the speaker rather than what is going on around them. Activity in the background can also be obscured with a virtual background image like a classroom or living room scene. This technique is particularly useful if you want to give the impression that everyone is in the same room. It is frequently used for corporate purposes such as remote meetings and training sessions but can also be used to promote family telepresence and limit what can be observed in areas behind the patient.

Technology Requirements

Successful family telepresence requires infrastructure that allows each party to clearly see and hear one another. Each party must have access to a:

1. Device with Internet connectivity or cellular service and sufficient processing speed and disk space to run a video chat application. In a hospital setting, this device must be mobile. Mobility is less of an issue for family or support persons where a stationary computer may serve their needs.
2. Microphone, preferably with noise-canceling properties, and the ability to pick up a person's voice from a distance.
3. Speaker with volume that is sufficient to be heard from a distance and over the other sounds that may occur in the clinical setting. Earbuds or headsets with an integrated microphone can be helpful if a patient is unable to hold a device close enough to be heard.
4. Webcam that can be centered on the patient's face and with enough digital resolution to work in low-light environments. Newer smartphones and tablets can automatically adapt to low light situations, and some smartphones have manual camera settings to accommodate low light.
5. Broadband Internet or cellular service with enough data available to support video chat.

Hardware used in the patient care setting must be able to be disinfected using standard methods for bedside electronic equipment. Use of earbuds and headsets with spongy ear or microphone coverings should be limited to a single individual if the ability to remove and disinfect those coverings is not possible. Ideally, hospital-supplied devices should have integrated systems that are Health Insurance Portability and Accountability Act (HIPAA) compliant and able to safeguard the security of protected patient information.

The pandemic presented challenges for maintaining privacy during patient communication. To address this, a limited waiver of HIPAA sanctions and penalties has been issued by the Department of Health and Human Services for hospitals operating under disaster protocols and liberalizes consent issues when communicating with family members or support persons involved in the patient's care.[16]

Technology Enhanced Family Presence: Our Hospital's Experience

Our 1157-bed academic medical facility, one of the largest public hospitals in the country, is located in an urban community and serves as the tertiary referral center for the state of Alabama and surrounding region. We care for a diverse population from across the Deep South that encompasses low-resource rural communities as well as affluent suburban and urban communities. Because of this, the personal devices patients and their families have available to them varies, as does their ability to use them. Access to cellular phone and Internet service also varies, particularly among families who live in rural or low resource areas.

Practices in promoting telepresence among patients, family, and health team members differed depending on the clinical setting. Before the pandemic, the supply of portable devices for video chat and video conferencing were adequate to meet the needs of patients who were separated from family or support persons. This was not the case after all patients admitted to the hospital relied on telepresence to engage with their loved ones. When patients did not have access to their own devices, many nurses and health team members responded by using their personal smartphones or tablets to engage patients with their family or support persons. In addition, hospital-owned tablets and telemedicine devices were recruited to this effort. These devices could be mounted to rolling carts to allow for hands-free operation, which was particularly helpful when patients could not hold and operate the device themselves.

Technical difficulties arose frequently and challenged nurses who found themselves instructing families on how to access the Internet and download and use video chat applications. This was particularly problematic for families in rural areas where the infrastructure for cellular and Internet service was limited and the usual options to connect to the Internet, like coffee shops and libraries, were closed.

No policy or procedures were in place to guide the duration of time digital resources could be used, number of times families could be contacted, aspects of care that were appropriate for video transmission, and when video transmission should have been limited. Other logistical challenges included:

- Difficulty in determining next of kin and code word use for release of HIPAA-protected information.
- Concern that using devices outside of a secure network might be vulnerable to breaches in privacy and hacking.
- Discomfort on the part of nurses who felt families might be using digital technology as surveillance of nursing activities rather than emotional support and patient interaction.

Nursing Presence

When virtual contact with families was not possible, nurses and other health team members attempted to fill the void by acting as surrogate support persons to their patients. Presence is defined by the NIC system as "being with another, both physically and psychologically, during times of need."[6] The focus of this intervention is on the nurse's physical and emotional presence with the patient. **Table 2** summarizes the key attitudes and activities that make up this nursing intervention.

Impact of COVID-19 on Nursing Presence

During COVID-19 surges, hospitals nationwide were challenged by reduced nursing staff because of illness, mandated quarantine, retirement, and resignation. Unfortunately, this occurred at a time when hospitals were closed to patients' families and there was an increased need for nursing presence as a surrogate support person.

As hospital censuses rose, the nurses' ability to be present physically and emotionally for their patients became strained. All hospital personnel wore face masks, but for nurses who practiced in settings that cared for COVID-19 patients, personal protective equipment (PPE) included gowns, gloves, face shields or goggles, and masks designed for advanced filtration such as N95 filtering facepiece respirators, and powered air-purifying respirators. These essential pieces of equipment altered the nurse's physical appearance by partially or wholly obscuring their face.

Our Hospital's Response

Our hospital's top priority during this acute nursing shortage was to ensure effective nursing presence by rapidly onboarding local nurses who may have chosen to step away from patient care or practice in non-inpatient settings. In addition, the hospital and School of Nursing established a collaborative effort called "The Helping Hands Program" that deployed School of Nursing faculty-led student teams to act as force multipliers and fill gaps in staffing or act as a potential source of sitters and patient social support. Although some faculty members worked individually, others supervised up to 10 students and assumed a variety of roles based on their clinical expertise. These roles included providing patient care in the ICU with a focus on placing and maintaining patients in the prone position, in-direct patient care activities, and support of staff nurses in areas with low staffing, and staffing vaccination clinics.

PPE, although critical to patient and nurse safety, wholly or partially obscures the patient's ability to see the nurse's face. Since facial expression is one of the ways that human beings communicate emotion, PPE can impair the nurse's ability to communicate their emotional availability to the patient. This non-verbal communication is essential to nursing presence. To bridge this gap, nursing staff attached their picture in the form of a large button to their PPE with the title, "this is the smile behind my mask." This low-tech approach was used to enhance nursing presence by allowing the patient to "see" the nurse's face.

Lessons Learned

Telepresence practices preceded policy in the early days of the pandemic, and this led to the ethical, technical, and logistical challenges discussed earlier. These challenges taught us valuable lessons in the large-scale use of telepresence as social support for our patients. These lessons are summarized in **Table 3**.

Although the pandemic presented many hardships to families and nurses, it also provided opportunities to rethink the meaning of family and nurse presence. The strategies used to facilitate presence for patients will continue to benefit future patients and families when their ability to be physically present with one another is limited by circumstances like distance, finances, and illness.

PRESENCE IN NURSING EDUCATION
The Community of Inquiry Framework

Although being present in a collaborative virtual environment is an emerging phenomenon in acute and critical care nursing practice, the concept has been used for more than two decades in education. Garrison and colleagues[17] proposed three types of presence that are essential to successful virtual collaborative learning in the Community of Inquiry model. Although the goal of virtual presence was critical thinking, this model provides insights for facilitating collaboration and connectedness within all communities of learning.

The Community of Inquiry framework identifies three dimensions of presence that are essential for learning in virtual environments: (1) *social presence*, or the ability to project one's own social and emotional self and perceive others as real people in virtual settings; (2) *teaching presence*, or the ability to design, implement, and successfully facilitate course activities to ensure learning; and (3) *cognitive presence*, or the extent to which learners are able to engage with course content to achieve higher-level thinking and learning.[18–20] These three elements combine in virtual environments to create a "community" that is a constructivist, interactive educational experience with identifiable content, climate, and discourse (**Fig. 1**).[17] Extensive research using this framework has shown that each dimension can be enhanced using various methods to improve learning outcomes and promote student satisfaction and engagement.[21]

Social presence. Social presence is the degree to which all members of the community participate in constructing new understandings and knowledge together. Building a community of learners can be challenging, as it requires communication, interaction,

Table 2		
Key attitudes and activities attributed to effective nurse presence[6]		
Attitudes	**Physical Activities**	**Psychosocial Activities**
Acceptance and empathy for the patient's experiences	Stay with the patient	Demonstrate availability to the patient
Desire to establish trust and provide positive regard	Provide reassuring touch when appropriate	Address anxiety and promote the patient's emotional and physical safety
Comfortable when patients do not give interactional responses	Lend assistance as a helper while supporting patient autonomy	Communicate understanding of the patient's experience
Cultural sensitivity and openness to patient traditions and beliefs	Offer to remain with the patient during initial interactions with other health team members	Listen to the patient's concerns
	Offer to contact other support persons (clergy, family, and others)	Use silence when appropriate
		Provide reassurance and support

and a sense of trust. Yet Garrison and colleagues[17] argue that social presence is essential for creating and sustaining the other two elements of the model, as learners must feel supported by their teachers and peers and willing to share experiences to collaborate for meaningful knowledge construction.

In practice, this interactive community often must be created and sustained within a short period of time. Virtual environments add another layer of complexity in that teachers and learners must be able to use technology effectively to delve into course material, apply concepts, and reflect on learning. Strategies to create a strong social presence include conducting synchronous class meetings, using icebreakers and other prompts to promote interaction, encouraging learners to share personal stories, and designing group assignments that require collaborative activities for problem-solving.[22,23]

Teaching presence. Garrison and colleagues[17] claim that a lack of strong teaching presence is usually the cause of failed educational experiences in virtual settings. Learners must have someone to organize, facilitate, and direct their learning by identifying appropriate course material and activities, sharing real-world applications, and providing valuable and timely feedback. Teachers must demonstrate expertise, not only in subject matter, but also in implementing strategies to support diverse learners in collaborative virtual learning communities.[24] These strategies might include providing regular announcements, creating videos to convey course material, responding to questions in detail and in a timely manner, adding to or redirecting discussions as needed, and providing extensive feedback on graded assignments.

Cognitive presence. Although the other two elements of this model involve participants, the element of cognitive presence is defined by Garrison and colleagues[17] as the extent to which these participants are "able to construct meaning through sustained communication" (2000, p. 89). They point out that this ability is key to achieving the ultimate educational goal: thinking critically.[25] Cognitive presence is therefore the most important element in the model, though it cannot be sustained without the presence of the other two. To achieve it, learners must demonstrate that they have developed higher-level thinking skills to solve problems, communicate effectively, link and apply facts and concepts, and even generate new ideas.

Table 3
Strategies for using telepresence as social support

Expected Challenge	Suggested Strategy
Ethical challenges	Develop guidelines for: 1. Steps to protect patient privacy during video chat sessions 2. Fair distribution of limited virtual communication technology 3. How and when video chat will be initiated 4. When to sensitively conclude a session to maintain the patient's dignity during nursing care
Technical challenges	Reduce confusion among staff and improve ease of use by: 1. Standardizing communication technology used at the bedside 2. Engaging Information Systems/Information Technology staff to support nurses and other health team members to use and trouble-shoot communication technology 3. Create a plan for coaching family and support persons in communication technology use
Logistical challenges	Provide staff development that prepares nurses and other health team members to facilitate family presence via video chat Inform the public of the options available to connect with hospitalized family members using video chat platforms Orient family members to expectations for video chat (identify who is present, recording prohibitions, time limits, and clinical reasons for ending the session) Determine who will monitor the session to ensure that patient privacy and dignity is maintained Use auxiliary personnel, like nursing and medical students, to initiate and monitor video chat sessions when nurses are not available

Impact of COVID-19 on Nursing Education

The abrupt onset of the COVID-19 pandemic in March 2020 hit most nursing schools in the middle of a semester. Courses being delivered in face-to-face settings had to be immediately converted to virtual platforms to ensure continued successful student progression in nursing programs. Although most nurse educators have some familiarity with using instructional technology, many had never taught in online courses before. In some cases, budget cuts forced administrators to dismiss adjunct instructors or teaching aides, leaving full-time faculty with increased workloads and more students to manage.

Students were also immediately impacted in terms of their educational trajectories. Many had to put off graduation due to course disruptions, illness, family challenges, or other hardships. Those who were able to continue in their nursing programs had to adjust to drastic changes in their educational experience. Many students had little practice in navigating virtual nursing courses in terms of technology, time management, and communication skills needed to be successful. Perhaps the most consequential threat to nursing students was that clinical courses were disrupted or suspended, denying many students access to practice vital patient care skills.

Impact of COVID-19 on Presence in Communities of Inquiry

The essential need for social, teaching, and cognitive presence in virtual courses was dramatically evident during the first few months of adjustment to changes brought on by the COVID-19 pandemic. Nursing students in some face-to-face courses with small enrollment numbers might have already experienced a strong sense of community

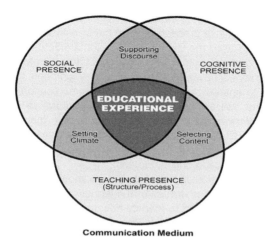

Communication Medium

Fig. 1. Community of inquiry framework. (*From* Garrison DR, Anderson T, Archer W. Critical Inquiry in a Text-Based Environment: Computer Conferencing in Higher Education. The Internet and Higher Education. 1999;2(2-3):87-105.)

and camaraderie that they could carry over to virtual settings, but many in other classes, especially those with large enrollments, felt immediately isolated. Many nurse educators struggled to implement strategies to facilitate collaborative activities and effective communication, often using learning management systems (LMSs) that they had previously used only as repositories or technologies that they had never been trained to use. Changes in course design and delivery methods required teachers and learners to engage with content in new ways, sometimes delaying essential educational activities or forcing faculty to change or delete them altogether. Of course, all stakeholders were affected at some level by the pandemic itself, causing various types of distress that inevitably disrupted cognitive presence among learners.

Educational researchers will be assessing the impact of these changes for years to come. However, numerous anecdotal accounts of these types of experiences during the pandemic highlight a need for a better understanding of how to build a strong presence in all three dimensions of the community of inquiry framework and integrate them effectively for successful nursing education, even in times of crisis.

Pivot to Virtual Learning: Our School's Experience

At our large research university, the shift to virtual learning across all bachelor's master's, and doctoral-level nursing programs required us to quickly implement broadly scaled initiatives designed to help faculty maintain a strong teaching presence. Fortunately, we already had an Office of Technology and Innovation within our school, with directors for instructional technology and instructional innovation and a dedicated instructional design team, including a videographer. To assist in the rapid transition of all courses to online delivery, this team increased opportunities for faculty training and support for technology and course design and delivery. They changed the monthly face-to-face instructional design training sessions to weekly virtual ones, and average attendance more than doubled as faculty eagerly sought assistance with Zoom technology features such as chat, breakout rooms, and virtual backgrounds to increase social presence. The instructional technology-focused Zoom sessions gave faculty real-time support as they quickly adjusted to virtual environments, and the archived sessions provided easily accessible resources to help faculty sustain teaching, social, and cognitive presence during the transition.

Though everyone had used the Canvas LMS to some extent, faculty delved further into how to create engaging content with a variety of activities to appeal to students with diverse learning styles, how to construct group assignments for virtual collaboration, and strategies to ensure clear, constructive communication. Our videographer demonstrated how to use a video cloud platform (Kaltura) to create and upload high-quality videos, allowing faculty to continue to sustain teaching presence. The team also taught faculty to use the video software GoReact, which provides a platform for faculty and students to upload and comment on videos, increasing possibilities for teaching and social presence in online courses.

Clinical courses were particularly challenging, as most students were prohibited from entering hospital settings for clinical instruction during the height of the pandemic. As a result, faculty had to identify how to use technology in new ways to conduct simulations and assess students' psychomotor skills for clinical care. Many faculty collaborated with our simulation staff and videographer to develop unfolding video case studies in which standardized patients and other participants enacted scenarios in clinical settings, stopping at intervals to ask students to make decisions regarding patient care. These simulations used human actors who were able to communicate emotion through facial expression and tone of voice, which contributed to the sense of human presence.

Some simulations relied on avatars to represent human beings, a practice that is popular in video games and online gaming communities. Avatars who represent human beings provide social presence in virtual interactions and people respond positively to avatars that have similarities to themselves.[26,27] Because of this, an effort was made to create avatars that represented people of both genders with varying skin tone, eye color, hairstyles, and clothing. In our undergraduate community/public health course, telepresence and avatars were combined to engage students in simulated disaster response and global health crisis scenarios. The goal of the simulations was to develop the students' prioritization and critical thinking skills by working in teams to triage disaster victims or address diseases of poverty with limited resources. Use of the Zoom video chat platform allowed students to work in teams to review patient information and determine a plan of action. The avatars were static and two-dimensional, which impacted their realism, but students reported that they were able to think of them as human beings in need of urgent care.

Many of the strategies we used to maintain a strong presence in virtual classes at the height of the pandemic were possible because we already had support staff and technologies in place. Though the abrupt transition caused tremendous stress and confusion initially, it forced us to be innovative and more flexible to keep all stakeholders motivated and connected. The challenges of the pandemic heightened our awareness of the need to continually develop new ways to sustain and improve teaching, social, and cognitive presence in our classes. Some of our solutions required additional resources, but in planning for the future, institutions with limited funding may consider less costly strategies to support presence in communities of inquiry. For example, faculty or students may use smartphones to record videos and then upload them to a discussion board for comments. Students may choose to use free applications such as Slack, GroupMe, or Microsoft Teams to organize their work for group assignments. In the absence of instructional designers, peer mentoring by more experienced faculty can help fill training and support needs. Through collaboration and ingenuity, faculty and students can devise ways to stay connected in virtual settings to promote higher level learning.

Table 4 Common challenges with presence during virtual nursing instruction		
Type of Presence	**Challenges**	**Potential Solutions**
Teaching	Faculty training and support	Maintain a skilled instructional design team, including a videographer to work with faculty to create course videos
		Implement regularly scheduled trainings for virtual course design and delivery
		Create peer mentoring initiatives for faculty to build skills and ensure consistency of course delivery and curriculum
Teaching, social	Familiarity with technology	Use learning management system consistently across programs in face-to-face and virtual courses
		Develop videos and simulations for virtual delivery
Teaching, social	Communication	Set expectations regarding class participation
		Model professional behavior and communication
		Adhere to a regular schedule of announcements
		Maintain a discussion board for general questions and comments about course content
Social	Collaboration in virtual settings	Design courses to include regular group/team assignments requiring students to collaborate to solve problems
		Provide information about platforms that can be used to collaborate in groups/teams
Social	Coping skills for mental health issues	Provide contact information for mental health counseling in all courses
		Discuss signs and symptoms of depression, anxiety, addiction, suicidal thoughts, etc. in appropriate courses and as needed
		Be flexible with deadlines, if possible, especially in times of crisis
		Invite expert speakers to discuss mental health issues with students, faculty, and staff
Cognitive	Diverse learning styles	Include a variety of learning activities in all courses
		When appropriate, allow students to demonstrate mastery in different ways

Lessons Learned

The pandemic challenged nurse educators to rethink traditional teaching strategies and in doing so taught valuable lessons for future nursing education program development and implementation. **Table 4** aligns types of presence with common challenges during virtual nursing instruction and potential solutions for each.

SUMMARY

Human presence is essential to nursing care and education. The physical presence of a person is only one means of being present to others. The COVID-19 pandemic has required nurses to facilitate human presence at the bedside and in the classroom by leveraging communication technology. Although using these technologies can be challenging, the skills developed during a time of urgent need will serve our patients and students well into the future.

CLINICS CARE POINTS

- Family and support persons are partners in patient care; supporting the presence of family and support persons is a nursing intervention.
- Nurses can use technology to establish telepresence when in-person family and support presence is not possible.
- Technology-enhanced family presence requires guidance by institutional policies regarding equipment and technical specifications, patient privacy, and general rules regarding technology use by patients and family.
- Staff development is essential in the preparation of nurses and other health team members to facilitate family presence via telepresence.
- The Community of Inquiry framework provides insight into creation of a virtual classroom environment where cognitive, teaching, and social presence support student learning.

DISCLOSURE

The authors have nothing to disclose.

REFERENCES

1. Sandford A. Coronavirus: half of humanity now on lockdown as 90 countries call for Confinement 2020. Available at: https://www.euronews.com/2020/04/02/coronavirus-in-europe-spain-s-death-toll-hits-10-000-after-record-950-new-deaths-in-24-hou.
2. Center NGSF. Environmental Impacts of the COVID-19 Pandemic, as Observed from Space. ScienceDaily 2020. Available at: https://www.sciencedaily.com/releases/2020/12/201208162957.htm.
3. Usher BM, Hill Kathleen M. AACN Practice Alert: Family Visitation in the Adult Intensive Care Unit. Crit Care Nurse 2016;36(1):e15–9. https://doi.org/10.4037/ccn2016677.
4. Voo TC, Senguttuvan M, Tam CC. Family Presence for Patients and Separated Relatives During COVID-19: Physical, Virtual, and Surrogate. J Bioethical Inq 2020;17(4):767–72.
5. Dokken D, Ahmann E. Family Presence During Challenging Times. Pediatr Nurs 2020;46(4):161–2.
6. Butcher HK, Bulecheck Gloria M, Dochterman Joanne M, et al. Nursing interventions Classification (NIC). 7th edition. Elsevier; 2018. p. 489.
7. Fumagalli S, Boncinelli L, Lo Nostro A, et al. Reduced Cardiocirculatory Complications With Unrestrictive Visiting Policy in an Intensive Care Unit. Circulation 2006;113(7):946–52.

8. Hupcey JE. Looking out for the patient and ourselves – the process of family integration into the ICU. J Clin Nurs (Wiley-blackwell) 1999;8(3):253–62.
9. Davidson JE, Powers K, Hedayat KM, et al. Clinical practice guidelines for support of the family in the patient-centered intensive care unit: American College of Critical Care Medicine Task Force 2004–2005. Crit Care Med 2007;35(2):605–22.
10. McAdam JL, Puntillo KA. Open visitation policies and practices in US ICUs: can we ever get there? Crit Care 2013;17(4):171.
11. CMS. Hospital Visitation – Phase II Visitation for Patients who are Covid-19 Negative. 2020. Available at: https://www.cms.gov/files/document/covid-hospital-visitation-phase-ii-visitation-covid-negative-patients.pdf. Accessed June 26 2020.
12. Control CfD. Interim Infection Prevention and Control Recommendations for Healthcare Personnel During the Coronavirus Disease 2019 (COVID-19) Pandemic. 2021. Available at: https://www.cdc.gov/coronavirus/2019-ncov/hcp/infection-control-recommendations.html. Accessed date September 10 2021.
13. Hajek A, König H-H. Social Isolation and Loneliness of Older Adults in Times of the COVID-19 Pandemic: Can Use of Online Social Media Sites and Video Chats Assist in Mitigating Social Isolation and Loneliness? Gerontology 2021;67(1):121–4.
14. Sherman WR, Craig Alan B. Understanding Virtual Reality: Interface, Application, and Design. In: The Morgan Kauffman Series in computer Graphics. 2 edition. Elsevier; 2018.
15. Groom LL, Brody, Abraham A, et al. Defining Telepresence as Experienced in Telehealth Encounters: A Dimensional Analysis. J Nurs Scholarship 2021;53(6):709–17.
16. U.S. Department of Health and Human Services. COVID-19 & HIPAA Bulletin: Limited Waiver of HIPAA Sanctions and Penalties During a Nationwide. Public Health Emergency 2020. https://www.hhs.gov/sites/default/files/hipaa-and-covid-19-limited-hipaa-waiver-bulletin-508.pdf.
17. Garrison DR, Anderson T, Archer W. Critical Inquiry in a Text-Based Environment: Computer Conferencing in Higher Education. Internet Higher Education 1999;2(2–3):87–105.
18. Boston W, Diaz SR, Gibson AM, et al. An exploration of the relationship between indicators of the Community of Inquiry framework and retention in online programs. J Asynchronous Learn Networks 2019;14(1):67–83.
19. Flock H. Designing a community of inquiry in online courses. Int Rev Res Open Distributed Learn 2020;21(1):134–52.
20. Lawa KMY, Gengb S, Lic T. Student enrollment, motivation and learning performance in a blended learning environment: The mediating effects of social, teaching, and cognitive presence. Comput Education 2019;136:1–12.
21. Sternbom S. A systematic review of the Community of Inquiry. Internet and Higher Education39 2018;22–32.
22. d'Alessio MA, Lundquist LL, Schwartz JJ, et al. Social presence enhances student performance in an online geology course but depends on instructor facilitation. J Geosci Education 2019;67(3):222–36.
23. Richardson JC, Maeda Y, Lv J, et al. Social presence in relation to students' satisfaction and learning in the online environment: A meta-analysis. Comput Hum Behav 2017;71:402–17.
24. Hambacher E, Ginn K, Slater K. From Serial Monologue to Deep Dialogue: Designing Online Discussions to Facilitate Student Learning in Teacher Education Courses. Action Teach Education 2018;40(3):239–52.

25. Garrison DR, Anderson T, Archer W. Critical thinking, cognitive presence, and computer conferencing in distance education. Am J Distance Education 2001; 15(1):7–23.
26. Barbier L, Fointiat V. To Be or Not Be Human-Like in Virtual World. Brief Research Report. Front Computer Sci 2020. https://doi.org/10.3389/fcomp.2020.00015.
27. Nowak K, Rauh C. The influence of the Avatar on Online Perceptions of Anthropomorphism, Androgyny, Credibility, Homophily, and Attraction. J Computer-Mediated Commun 2006;11:153–78.

Student Response Systems in Online Nursing Education

Elizabeth Hutson, PhD, APRN-CNP, PMHNP-BC

KEYWORDS

- Audience response system • Clicker • Distance education • Gamification
- Mobile applications • Student engagement • Smartphone
- Student response system

KEY POINTS

- Active learning and student engagement with course content, peers, and instructor are critical in online nursing education.
- Student response systems (SRSs) can promote student engagement and encourage critical thinking to during synchronous online classes.
- Instructors need to consider barriers related to cost and technological issues when implementing SRSs in their online classroom.

INTRODUCTION

Nursing instructors are challenged with creating meaningful learning experiences that spark student engagement. Student engagement has been defined as the quality of effort on the part of the student or how much the student is involved in educational tasks.[1] Passive learning (for example, when students sit in a classroom listening to instructors lecture) does not inspire student engagement. In contrast, active learning results in better learning outcomes than passive learning and encourages students to actively and intentionally engage in the learning process.[2,3]

The use of active learning strategies in nursing education is supported by professional nursing organizations such as the American Association of Colleges of Nursing (AACN).[4] The National League for Nursing (NLN) is committed to faculty excellence in using emerging technologies to advance the health of the nation.[5] Using active learning strategies in the classroom helps students progress from the lower levels of Bloom's Taxonomy, where the focus is on remembering information, to higher levels of learning that involve application and evaluation.[6] Interactive learning techniques encourage students to practice critical thinking skills, which are especially important

Texas Tech University Health Sciences Center, School of Nursing, 3601 4th Street, Lubbock, TX 79430, USA
E-mail address: Elizabeth.Hutson@ttuhsc.edu

Nurs Clin N Am 57 (2022) 539–549
https://doi.org/10.1016/j.cnur.2022.06.004
0029-6465/22/© 2022 Elsevier Inc. All rights reserved.

nursing.theclinics.com

in health science fields where students need to perform at the highest level of Bloom's taxonomy, with application of skills in clinical practice.

The use of active learning strategies is critical to student engagement in online coursework. Student response systems (SRSs) can be used in online nursing courses to promote active learning and engage students in the learning process. Although SRSs are not new in traditional classrooms, their use in online courses increased during the COVID-19 pandemic when many courses were rapidly transitioned to an online format. Although some instructors are concerned about students using their personal devices, such as laptops, cell phones, and tablets, in class because of the distraction they are presumed to cause,[7] the reality is that students already have multiple devices at their fingertips and are using them during class despite faculty objections.[8] Therefore, the instructors have a compelling opportunity to use the devices students already have in their hands to enhance education rather than compete with the distraction students' devices may cause.

This article provides an overview of SRSs in nursing education, focusing on their implementation in online synchronous coursework. SRSs provide a method for instructors to promote active learning and student engagement with the course content, their classmates, and the instructor. Benefits of using SRSs in nursing education include student engagement through gamification, motivation to complete pre-class preparation work, and development of critical thinking skills. Potential challenges to using SRSs in the online classroom include cost and technological issues. Recommendations for implementation of SRSs and an example of how an SRS was used in a graduate nursing course for a large-group simulation debriefing are discussed.

BACKGROUND

Although SRSs are popular in health science education, there is limited research specifically addressing SRS effects on learning outcomes in nursing education. A qualitative review of undergraduate nursing students' perceptions of SRSs revealed that students perceived the SRS positively, specifically mentioning benefits such as improved learning, formative assessment opportunities, and increased participation.[9] Formative assessment, where the instructor monitors student learning and provides feedback in a low-stakes environment, has been found to be an important learning strategy. Formative assessment allows students to see how others are doing and also prompts discussion on concepts that were not clear. A study found that SRSs work to improve assessment and increase attendance and interactions between students and instructors.[10] SRSs have been found to be especially beneficial in large-enrollment classes in which students typically would not be able to interact easily with other students or the instructor.[11]

In a study of undergraduate and graduate nursing students, frequency of student use of an SRS was compared with students' final grades.[12] Although a strong relationship was not found in every course, likely due to variations in the implementation of the SRS, the researchers found that students who responded more frequently to SRS prompt had higher final grades in an undergraduate pathophysiology course. Specifically, for every response the student submitted to the SRS, their final grade increased by 0.25 (out of 100). The authors discussed the importance of requiring student participation in SRS activities rather than making participation optional as a key factor in improving final grades for the greatest number students in a course. Furthermore, instructors received positive feedback from students when the SRS was used in synchronous classes, where immediate feedback, rationales, and elaboration were provided.[12]

Student Response Systems

There are many types of active learning strategies, such as role playing and unfolding case studies.[13] SRSs, also known as audience response systems, personal response systems, or clicker systems, are another way to facilitate active learning. SRSs allow the instructor to present course content, ask questions to the class, and see the students' answers in real time (**Fig. 1**). In both online and in-person classroom settings, the instructor uses an SRS to present course content to students, and students respond using their computer or mobile device (typically a smartphone or tablet). The student responses are received by the SRS software, aggregated, and displayed in a table, chart, or graph so the instructor can share the collective results and correct answers back to the class. Ultimately, the aggregated student responses help the instructor know if students are comprehending the material, and they also help the student engage in self-assessment and reflection to determine if they are on the right track in their learning. This process results in audience-paced instruction, meaning that student comprehension is driving the learning. Most SRSs allow the instructor to choose from a variety of question types including multiple choice, multiple select,

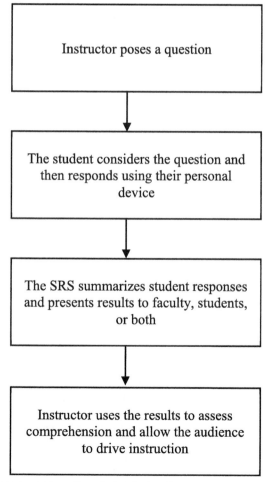

Fig. 1. Student response system flow during instruction.

short answer, matching, polling, drawing, and more. Although these types of questions have been used for rapid self-assessment in traditional classrooms for decades (for example, a student responds to an in-class prompt on paper and hands the paper to the instructor), SRSs allow student responses to be collected digitally, analyzed quickly, and stored online so the instructor can review the assessment results either immediately, during class, or after class, with or without informing the students of the results. There are many free, partially free, and proprietary SRSs, including Nearpod TopHat, UniDoodle, Echo360, OMBEA, Poll Everywhere, Via Response, Turning Technologies, Infuse Learning, Socrative, iClickers, Kahoot! , Quiz Socket, each with unique specifications that make them well suited for certain types of courses and classroom contexts.

An important concern to address in implementing an SRS is student ownership of mobile devices and the ability to learn and use the new technology. Fortunately, most research has found smartphone, tablet, or laptop ownership to be largely ubiquitous, especially among university students. According to 2018 data from the NLN, 50% of doctoral-level nursing students, nearly 83% of master's-level students, and 97% of bachelor's-level students are under the age of 40.[14] Thus, the majority of nursing students are under the age of 40 and can be considered "digital natives." Digital natives grew up with the Internet and speak the language of computers.[15] When these students come to the educational setting, they expect to use technology in the classroom. With nearly 95% of individuals ages 18–49 years owning a smartphone,[16] most nursing students are ready to use SRSs in the nursing classroom. It would be prudent for instructors to ask students before beginning SRS activities whether they have their own mobile device that they are willing to use for class and be prepared to provide technical support or have tech-support contact information ready. Although SRSs provide an engaging approach to teaching and learning, instructors need to design their instruction thoughtfully and integrate the technology into active classrooms while considering the potential challenges.

Using SRSs in nursing education can enhance student engagement in online courses, especially those that include synchronous components. Furthermore, asking students to use their mobile devices to engage in active learning can be an effective instructional strategy even when students are learning remotely and on their own schedule. An important first step for instructors in the implementation of SRSs in the online classroom is understanding the benefits this technology offers and being prepared to deal with challenges that may arise.

ROLE OF STUDENT RESPONSE SYSTEMS IN ONLINE STUDENT ENGAGEMENT

Student engagement in both in-person and online courses is challenging. Online synchronous classrooms, where students may or may not have their cameras turned on, pose a unique and significant challenge. There are three main types of student engagement: (1) student engagement with course content, (2) student engagement with their classmates, and (3) student engagement with instructors. **Table 1** presents an overview of potential barriers to each type of engagement. All three types of engagement are critical for student achievement of learning outcomes.

Lack of student engagement was especially problematic in the beginning of the COVID-19 pandemic, when students reported lack of social interactions with classmates and the instructor in online courses.[11] Not surprisingly, students agreed that social interactions play a positive role in their learning outcomes and wellbeing. Students need to feel connected to the instructors and their peers to connect effectively with instructional content.[17] In online nursing education, integration of active learning

Table 1		
Barriers to student engagement in online courses		
Barriers to Engagement with Course Content	**Barriers to Engagement with Classmates**	**Barriers to Engagement with Instructors**
• Low motivation or lack of time to complete prep work before class • Student confusion on important topics with general perception of lack of time for faculty to clarify • Students focus on information recall and struggle to move to higher levels of learning and critical thinking • Technical issues and anxiety related to use of learning technologies • Long periods of lecture in nursing courses (to allow for clinical days) means students are subject to "Zoom fatigue"	• Lack of interpersonal connections with other students • Uncertainty about how to project individual personalities • No time before, after, or during class for students to connect naturally • Student isolation, which can lead to burnout and course drop/fail/withdrawal • Instructor is unfamiliar with importance of peer-to-peer learning and strategies to engage students with their peers	• Instructors struggle to let their personality and teaching style show during online courses • Instructors miss student confusion or are unaware of which concepts students are struggling with the most • Tension between time spent engaging with students vs troubleshooting technological issues • Students struggle to speak up or communicate effectively with instructors during online courses

strategies is not optional. Rather, best practice in learning design requires active learning strategies to support student success. SRSs offer a range of opportunities for instructors to promote active learning and engagement in synchronous online instruction.

SRSs provide a way to engage students with course content, peers, and their instructor, and they promote active learning by enhancing participation and providing students and their instructor with feedback in real time.[18] SRSs increase student attention levels and promote interaction between students and the instructor.[19] SRSs encourage everyone in the class to respond to questions posed by the instructor, rather than relying on a few students who are brave enough to speak up in class. Although instructors use SRSs in different ways, there are common instructional approaches, such as gamification, pre-class preparation requirements, and critical thinking activities that optimize the benefits of implementing an SRS in an online nursing course.

Gamification

One of the inherent components of an SRS is gamification. Gamification in education has been defined as "the introduction of game design elements and gameful experiences in the design of learning processes."[20] Gamification is not new to digital natives; it is prevalent in many apps where tokens, coins, and other rewards are earned for participation and engagement with the app. Gamification is used in SRSs when the instructor poses a question and students earn points by answering quickly or correctly. Even when there are no points involved, students are naturally inclined to engage in friendly competition with peers. Gamification raises the stakes for participation and can promote student motivation, which is an important concept in student achievement.[21] Importantly, the participation, engagement, and competition generated by an SRS can make the learning experience fun.

Another important feature in SRSs is the option for anonymous participation. A common concern about student participation in class is fear of saying an incorrect answer and subsequent embarrassment in front of peers.[22,23] In SRSs, the student can enter their real name or a fake name if the instructor allows it. Regardless of whether real or fake student names are used, the instructor chooses to show or hide names to protect student confidentiality, and students who might otherwise stay silent in a traditional verbal classroom discussion do not have to worry that their peers will witness them answering a question incorrectly. For example, when a multiple-choice question is presented to students in Nearpod, the instructor can see each student's individual response, but Nearpod also compiles all student responses so the instructor can share them immediately, as a collection of answers, with the entire class. When a short-answer question is presented in Nearpod, again, the instructor can see every individual student's response and can even share an individual response with the class, but the student's name is hidden from students when it is shared. This is an important benefit of SRSs as the instructor no longer needs to rely on a few students who feel comfortable speaking up in class to generate open discussions. SRSs allow for audience-paced instruction and maximum participation by every student in the class, rather than instructor-paced instruction driven by a few students who are more outspoken than their classmates.[24]

Motivation to Complete Pre-Class Preparation Work

Another way that SRSs can promote student engagement with the course content is by requiring pre-class preparation work in a flipped-classroom approach. Students engage in pre-class learning activities in advance, such as listening to pre-recorded lectures or completing required readings. Then, their knowledge of the course content is tested using an SRS during the time they spend in class. This strategy encourages students to engage independently with the course content before class and then come to class prepared to test their critical thinking skills.[25] Although it is common for instructors to assign pre-class preparation work, it can be challenging to motivate students to complete this work. Ensuring students understand that their knowledge will be tested during class helps motivate them to come to class prepared.

Critical Thinking Activities

When instructors use only passive learning strategies, students get stuck in the lower levels of learning according to Bloom's Taxonomy,[26] relying simply on recall and remembering information to show achievement of learning goals. Although recall is an important first step in meeting higher-level learning outcomes, nurse educators want students to be able to show more complex skills such as critique and evaluation in didactic settings, so they feel prepared to apply these skills in the clinical setting. SRSs can help promote critical thinking processes such as application, analysis, and evaluation using higher-level questions.[6,27] Consider, for example, a pharmacology course for which students have completed the preparation work by reading course content and listening to pre-recorded lectures to learn about medication. During class time, using an SRS, the instructor could pose a multiple-choice question, and students will select a medication they feel is appropriate for a particular case or scenario. Responding to this type of question would be categorized as *application* in Bloom's Taxonomy. The instructor would then receive immediate feedback from the SRS regarding which medications the students selected and thereby have real-time information about whether the students are comprehending the topic at hand and know whether to proceed on to the next concept or stop and provide remediation. The instructor might then choose to use a peer-instruction strategy by dividing

Table 2 Strategies to resolve barriers to student engagement with SRSs		
Student Engagement with Course Content	**Student Engagement with Classmates**	**Student Engagement with Instructors**
• Increase motivation to complete prep work • Use class time to actively test critical thinking skills • Guide students to achieve higher levels of learning • Employ principles of gamification • Provide interactive learning opportunities to support full attention and participation in long classes	• Students choose their own nicknames or icons • SRS results show students in real time whether peers are also struggling with the course content (or not) which helps ease anxiety • SRS results reveal the variety of answers peers select and show to students the importance of diversity of thought • SRSs can introduce difficult concepts that lead to peer instruction and critical thinking activities	• Instructors can use a variety of question types to engage students • Instructors can use wellness checks to ensure attendance and attention in the beginning, middle, and at the end of class • Instructors can assess in real time which concepts students are struggling with and spend more time focusing on that content

students into pairs and sending them to a breakout room in the online classroom platform to discuss with their peer the medication they selected, side-effect profile and dosing, and then, after students return to the large group, ask the same question a second time to see how responses change. This interactive peer discussion exercise would be categorized at the level of *analysis* in Bloom's Taxonomy. Although this approach is already in use in many courses, an instructional difference with a potentially meaningful impact on student learning is introduced by using an SRS. The SRS software collects student responses, and when the instructor chooses to share results, all students can visualize the answers their peers selected in real time. This strategy works especially well to stimulate discussion between peers and the instructor when there is more than one correct answer, and it provides students with opportunities to develop reasoning and argumentation skills.[28]

Although SRSs facilitate gamification, preparation work, and critical thinking to achieve higher levels of learning, there are many other ways SRSs can resolve challenges to student engagement. **Table 2** presents a summary of instructional approaches and strategies for using SRSs in online synchronous classes. An example of how an SRS was implemented in an online graduate nursing course for synchronous virtual simulation debriefing is presented in **Box 1**.

RECOMMENDATIONS FOR STUDENT RESPONSE SYSTEMS IN THE ONLINE CLASSROOM

There are many important considerations for implementing SRSs into a synchronous online classroom setting. Instructors should consider which SRS platforms, if any, are supported by their institution or used in other courses their students' curriculum. It is possible students have already been using an SRS in another course. It is much easier for an individual instructor to learn how to use a specific SRS than to ask a large group of students to learn to use a new SRS. Established SRS technology use at the institution may reduce costs and facilitate use and support of the SRS for students. Although

---

Box 1
Example of student response system use during online simulation debrief

Students in an online graduate-level Psychiatric Mental Health Nurse Practitioner (PMHNP) program completed individual objective structured clinical evaluations (OSCEs) as part of a clinical course. Approximately 50 students completed the OSCE via telehealth technology, with one instructor sitting in on each student's OSCE. Students completed pre-simulation activities to familiarize themselves with the patient (a suicidal adolescent with a history of depression) and were then given 30 minutes to complete the patient encounter. At the end of the 30-min patient encounter, the student and instructor debriefed for 10 minutes.

Then, during the next synchronous online class, students (n = 45) debriefed as a class using Nearpod. Faculty determined that using an SRS to debrief as a group was necessary because of the large class size and practical challenges in asking every student to share their individual debrief. Instructors created multiple-choice and short-answer questions and led students in a large-group debriefing.

Selected debriefing questions:
• What went well?
• What was the hardest part?
• Have you seen a patient present like this in your clinical or work setting?
• What was your greatest "take away" moment?
• Were you concerned her antidepressant was causing the suicidal ideation? How could you help determine this?
• What are some screening tools you can use to assess for suicidality in adolescents?

During the synchronous online class in Zoom, the instructor asked each question, stopping to share aggregate student responses to multiple-choice question, which led to more in-depth discussions. For example, the yes/no question "Were you concerned her antidepressant was causing the suicidal ideation?" led to an in-depth discussion of the Federal Drug Administration Black Box warning about risk of suicidal ideation with antidepressants and how to assess for this. By using an SRS to facilitate the debriefing activity, the instructor was also able to share individual student responses with the class, such as "I've never seen a case like this in my clinicals, but I've heard about it happening in practice so I'm glad I was able to practice." Student names were hidden when sharing responses to keep responses confidential. Comments such as this one led to deeper discussions about similar scenarios in practice and approaches to dealing with them. Ultimately, this large online group debrief allowed:
• The instructor to clarify and describe the expected outcome for the patient encounter.
• The instructor to ensure that each student fully participated in the debrief.
• The students to feel a sense of relief in that they all had similar anxieties leading up to and during the OSCE.
• The students to hear the instructors' descriptions of this type of encounter in their own clinical settings, which was particularly rich with 5 faculty members sharing their clinical stories with the entire class rather than small clinical groups or individual students.

---

some SRSs are free, or free with certain limitations, the cost of an SRS can be a prohibitive factor in implementation. If cost is a barrier that cannot be overcome, explore the features and limitations (often explained on comparison of pricing plans on vendor Web sites) of SRSs that offer a free version such as Kahoot or Nearpod.

Instructors should also consider whether they want to associate points or a grade with the SRSs activities. Getting students to participate in SRS activities can be a challenge when there is no association between their participation and their grade.[12]

Lastly, the potential for technological issues should not be understated, but as SRS technology continues to improve and the proportion of nursing students who are comfortable with technology steadily increases, problems with learning technologies become easier to solve. Most proprietary SRSs provide extensive technical troubleshooting documentation and support online, which is available for all users. Users

---

Box 2
Recommendations for SRS implementation

- Consider which SRSs may already be in use at your institution, and determine if a university, department, or individual course license is required to use a specific SRS in your course.
- Consider whether an SRS has already been used in your students' previous coursework; familiarity with technology supports quicker implementation and greater comfort levels.
- Consider potential cost of an SRS to the student; if they can use the SRS in subsequent courses, cost can be decreased.
- Find out whether the SRS you would like to use provides assessment and scoring reports for grading purposes and if the system can be integrated with your learning management system.
- Consider potential technical issues in advance and have a backup plan for students with individual challenges such as lack of a mobile device, technology problems, or accessibility concerns.
- Remember to leverage the SRS to teach. Be sure to add *content* in addition to *questions*.
- If grades are assigned for SRS participation, consider basing the grade on completeness of responses versus correct answers, which aligns with best practices in formative assessment.
- Use a variety of question types, including multiple-choice, board certification-type questions and short-answer, critical thinking application question.
- Add check-in type questions, unrelated to course content, in the middle of class sessions to assess for student attention and check in on the student's wellness. For example, "what is one thing you've done for your own wellness this week?"

---

who purchase licenses are typically provided with direct technical support for students and instructors by the vendor. Nevertheless, instructors should consider potential issues that may arise and plan accordingly. Alternative assignments or allowing students to complete SRS activities asynchronously are effective solutions for unexpected problems. Additional recommendations for SRS implementation are listed in **Box 2**.

SUMMARY

SRSs can be used effectively in online nursing education to promote student engagement with course content, their peers, and the instructor. There are many things to consider when implementing SRSs into online education, such as cost and technological issues, but with careful planning, SRSs can provide a rich educational experience involving active learning. SRSs encourage student engagement in the instructional process regardless of their perception of ability or self-confidence, which in turn supports inclusion and student-driven instruction. SRSs can provide an innovative way to assess student achievement of nursing competencies through the active demonstration of critical thinking skills.

CLINICS CARE POINTS

- Active learning and student engagement with course content, peers, and the instructor are critical to student success in online nursing education.
- Student response systems (SRSs) promote student engagement and active learning for students in online synchronous classrooms.

- SRSs facilitate audience-paced instruction and encourage participation by all students in class activities.
- SRS applications are available for use by educators and offer a wide range of features and levels of cost.
- Instructors need to carefully consider strategies to mitigate potential burdens of cost and technological issues for students when implementing SRSs.

DISCLOSURE

E. Hutson reports no financial interests or potential conflicts of interest.

REFERENCES

1. Pace CR. Achievement and the Quality of Student Effort. 1982.
2. Freeman S, Eddy SL, McDonough M, et al. Active learning increases student performance in science, engineering, and mathematics. Proc Natl Acad Sci 2014; 111(23):8410–5.
3. Styers ML, Van Zandt PA, Hayden KL. Active learning in flipped life science courses promotes development of critical thinking Skills. CBE—Life Sci Educ 2018;17(3). https://doi.org/10.1187/cbe.16-11-0332.
4. [AACN] AAoCoN. AACN's Vision for Academic Nursing. 2019. Available at: https://www.aacnnursing.org/Portals/42/News/White-Papers/Vision-Academic-Nursing.pdf. Accessed January 12, 2022.
5. National League for Nursing. A vision for the changing faculty role: preparing students for the technological world of health care. NLN Visions Series; 2015.
6. Davoudi M, Sadeghi NA. A systematic review of research on questioning as a high-level cognitive strategy. English Lang Teach 2015;8(10):76–90.
7. Flanigan AE, Babchuk WA. Digital distraction in the classroom: exploring instructor perceptions and reactions. Teach higher Educ 2020;1–19. https://doi.org/10.1080/13562517.2020.1724937.
8. Gallegos C, Nakashima H. Mobile devices: a distraction, or a useful tool to engage nursing students? J Nurs Educ 2018;57(3):170–3.
9. Sheng R, Goldie CL, Pulling C, et al. Evaluating student perceptions of a multi-platform classroom response system in undergraduate nursing. Nurse Educ Today 2019;78:25–31.
10. Petrucco C. Student Response Systems as a successful tool for formative assessment? Ital J Educ Res 2019;257–66.
11. Patterson B, Kilpatrick J, Woebkenberg E. Evidence for teaching practice: the impact of clickers in a large classroom environment. Nurse Educ Today 2010; 30(7):603–7.
12. Tornwall J, Lu L, Xie K. Frequency of participation in student response system activities as a predictor of final grade: an observational study. Nurse Educ Today 2020;87:104342.
13. Abeysekera L, Dawson P. Motivation and cognitive load in the flipped classroom: definition, rationale and a call for research. Higher Educ Res Dev 2015; 34(1):1–14.
14. National League for Nursing. Proportion of student enrollment by age and program type. Washington, DC: Biennial Survey of Schools of Nursing; 2018.
15. Prensky M. Digital natives, digital immigrants. On the Horizon MCB Press; 2001.

16. Mobile Fact Sheet. 2021. Available at: https://www.pewresearch.org/internet/fact-sheet/mobile/. Accessed January 12, 2022.
17. Almendingen K, Morseth MS, Gjølstad E, et al. Student's experiences with online teaching following COVID-19 lockdown: a mixed methods explorative study. PloS one 2021;16(8):e0250378.
18. Dangel HL, Wang CX. Student response systems in higher education: moving beyond linear teaching and surface learning. J Educ Technol Dev exchange 2008;1(1):8.
19. Collins J. Audience response systems: technology to engage learners. J Am Coll Radiol 2008;5(9):993–1000.
20. Dichev C, Dicheva D. Gamifying education: what is known, what is believed and what remains uncertain: a critical review. Int J Educ Technol higher Educ 2017; 14(1):1–36.
21. Linehan C, Kirman B, Lawson S, Chan G. Practical, appropriate, empirically-validated guidelines for designing educational games. presented at: Proceedings of the SIGCHI Conference on Human Factors in Computing Systems; 07 May 2011; Vancouver, BC, Canada. https://doi.org/10.1145/1978942.1979229.
22. Weaver RR, Qi J. Classroom Organization and Participation: College Students' Perceptions. J higher Educ 2005;76(5):570–601.
23. Atlantis E, Cheema BS. Effect of audience response system technology on learning outcomes in health students and professionals: an updated systematic review. Int J Evid Based Healthc 2015;13(1):3–8.
24. Walsh JA, Sattes BD. Quality questioning research-based practice to engage every learner. 2nd edition. Thousand Oaks, CA: Corwin; 2016.
25. Turner L, Keeler C. Should we prelab? A student-centered look at the time-honored tradition of prelab in clinical nursing education. Nurse educator 2015; 40(2). https://doi.org/10.1097/NNE.0000000000000095.
26. Anderson LW, Krathwohl DR. A taxonomy for learning, teaching, and assessing: a revision of bloom's taxonomy of educational objectives. Upper Saddle River, NJ: Addison Wesley Longman, Inc.; 2001.
27. Abrahamson A. A brief history of networked classrooms: effects, cases, pedagogy, and implications. audience response systems in higher education: applications and cases. 2006:1-25. doi:10.4018/978-1-59140-947-2.ch001.
28. Knight JK, Brame CJ. Peer Instruction. CBE—Life Sci Educ 2018;17(2). https://doi.org/10.1187/cbe.18-02-0025.

Influence of Technology in Supporting Quality and Safety in Nursing Education

Gerry Altmiller, EdD, APRN, ACNS-BC, ANEF, FAAN[a],*,
Loraine Hopkins Pepe, PhD, RN, NPD-BC, CCRN-K[b]

KEYWORDS

- Distance education • Educational technology • Innovation • Professional education
- Quality of health care • Patient safety • Simulation

KEY POINTS

- The COVID-19 pandemic and the subsequent need for social distancing accelerated the adoption of technology-driven strategies for work meetings on video platforms and use of quick response codes for just-in-time training.
- During the COVID-19 pandemic, technology was an essential tool for nursing professional development practitioners in the training of nurses that were redeployed to in-patient care units and for education on new drugs and protocols used to combat the virus.
- The innovation and resolve of nurses adapting technology to meet educational needs during the COVID-19 pandemic confirmed that accelerated change does not have to compromise quality and safety.

INTRODUCTION

The influence of nurses continues to grow as they positively impact care at the bedside with patients and families and in the larger society where the profession of nursing continues to be among the most trusted.[1] The COVID-19 pandemic illuminated the dedication of nurses providing direct care to patients but also highlighted the high degree of innovation and problem-solving skills nurses possess as they worked within an overburdened system in real-time, providing cutting-edge care as it was being discovered, and stretching resources beyond what was imaginable. Nurses quickly adjusted processes and adapted new protocols for delivering safe, high-quality care.

The authors have nothing to disclose.
No funding sources provided for this work.
[a] The College of New Jersey, School of Nursing and Health Sciences, 2000 Pennington Road, Ewing, NJ 08628, USA; [b] Jefferson-Einstein Healthcare Network, Nursing Education and Professional Development Department, 5501 Old York Road, Philadelphia, PA 19141, USA
* Corresponding author.
E-mail address: altmillg@tcnj.edu

Nurs Clin N Am 57 (2022) 551–562
https://doi.org/10.1016/j.cnur.2022.06.005
0029-6465/22/© 2022 Elsevier Inc. All rights reserved.

nursing.theclinics.com

The COVID-19 pandemic was the great equalizer among nurses. Where seasoned nurses frequently guide newer nurses in managing care and learning unit protocols, all nurses faced the same steep learning curve to quickly understand detailed procedures for triaging the care of patients with COVID-19, follow unfamiliar treatment modalities, and manage resources while adhering to strict isolation protocols. The rapid and continual change ever present in health care was accentuated by the emergent needs of a society in crisis, and nurses along with all health care professionals were challenged to find innovative solutions to deliver high-quality, safe care to patients. Technology played a significant role in supporting that work.

QUALITY AND SAFETY COMPETENCY IN PROFESSIONAL DEVELOPMENT

Since the call to improve health care from the Institute of Medicine (IOM; now the National Academy of Medicine) and the development of Quality and Safety Education for Nurses (QSEN), nurses have assumed a greater role in ensuring the quality and safety of patient care. The competencies identified by the IOM[2] and further developed by QSEN called for a new identity for nurses that demonstrated knowledge, skills, and attitudes that emphasized person-centered care, teamwork and collaboration, use of evidence-based practice, quality improvement skills, and the integrated use of informatics and technology in the provision of care for patients.[3] The American Association of Colleges of Nursing adopted those competencies in the development of *The Essentials: Core Competencies for Professional Nursing Education*,[4] which now serves as the roadmap for competency-based education for nurses to provide a stronger bridge to practice in developing competent practice-ready nurses. The inclusion of these competencies in nursing education provides standardized structure for content development and assessment in the teaching-learning process in prelicensure nursing education programs so that all students can expect the same education and all employers can expect the same competencies from their new hires.

The integration of quality and safety into education offerings in both practice and academia places a stronger emphasis on *why* interventions are necessary and not just *how* to complete a skill. For nursing professional development (NPD) practitioners, quality and safety competencies provide a structured, standardized process for developing education, shifting the focus from teaching tasks to teaching concepts about how to impact and promote high-quality, safe care.[5] Continuing education offerings, in-service programs, nursing orientation programs, and Transition to Practice programs remain integral processes in ensuring the competency of nurses in practice and come with a new reliance on technology as many health care settings shifted during the COVID-19 pandemic to online classes and virtual experiential learning. Not only has the setting for learning changed, but the education itself has shifted to include competency with informatics and health care technologies.

TECHNOLOGY'S INFLUENCE ON QUALITY AND SAFETY

As prominent as quality and safety have been in the evolution of nursing education, so has been the integration of informatics and health care technologies. Educational technologies including simulation and virtual simulation have created opportunities to emphasize and apply quality and safety competencies and have been instrumental in fostering a quality and safety mindset in nursing.[6] Data drives practice, and the measurement of nursing sensitive indicators is now commonplace on patient care units. In the practice setting, NPD practitioners use dashboard data to identify needed continuing education based on performance reports that indicate areas where benchmarks are not being met and improvement is needed.

Nurses will need to develop expertise at all levels of education and practice in applying data to support national quality initiatives aimed at improving access to care as well as management of care. The *Future of Nursing Report 2020–2030* calls for health care systems to employ nurses with expertise in technology to use digital platforms, artificial intelligence, and other technological innovations to address social determinants of health and health equity.[7] Training for these skills must begin in pre-licensure nursing education programs and be further supported in practice settings and advanced practice education if nurses are to appropriately use technology as not only a vehicle for learning but also a means for impacting the quality and safety of patient care.

TECHNOLOGY IN TEACHING AND LEARNING

The use of technology in all sectors continues to expand, significantly influencing the delivery of health care and the provision of health care education. The use of tablets and e-books rather than textbooks makes it possible for learners to have extended access to rapidly updated information. Active teaching strategies using technology to enhance learning have replaced outdated, stagnant methods from the past. These strategies support the engagement of the learner and promote adult learning principles of being self-directed, experiential, relevant, and problem-centered.[8] Learner engagement is essential to knowledge and skill development as it has been linked to the enhanced retention and application of knowledge in the clinical setting.[9]

To meet the learning needs of contemporary nurses, the professional development paradigm is shifting from using traditional approaches in teaching to using interactive educational technologies.[10,11] The result has been the infusion of innovative, creative, technology-focused teaching methods into curricula in both academic and practice settings. Although lectures, modules, and in-services have been the mainstay of nursing continuing education, the use of educational technology is now seen as an essential component in creating effective and engaging programs to enhance problem-solving, strengthen clinical judgment, and build skill application.[12]

DISCUSSION OF BEST PRACTICES FOR TEACHING QUALITY AND SAFETY USING TECHNOLOGY IN HEALTH CARE SETTINGS
Gaming

Gamification, or game-based learning, is an active learning strategy which uses a game to test the knowledge and skills of participants as they move toward achieving specific learning objectives. Game-based learning has been found to effectively enhance engagement with the added benefit of providing learners with immediate feedback.[12–14] As a teaching strategy, gaming meets the learning needs of many, especially members of Generation Z (those born after 1995) who are thought to be digitally native learners, as they often require interactive strategies to foster motivation, confidence, and judgment skills.[14]

Game-based learning is an approach whereby game elements are applied to nongame situations. A game model is chosen to serve as the template; these may include board games like Bingo, or popular electronic games such as Kahoot. Kahoot is a free online quizzing tool that can easily be used to assess learners' knowledge about topics such as dysrhythmia interpretation and management, wound assessment and staging, and medication administration practices. Educators insert the content which is presented as a quiz to learners who then select answers via their mobile device. After students select the answer from the choices, correct answers and aggregated response results from participants are displayed on the quiz screen.

Broadly familiar games such as *Jeopardy!* or *Who Wants to Be a Millionaire?* can be downloaded in an electronic template format for educational gaming. Instead of trivia content, instructional content is inserted in the template to meet learning objectives. These games are guided by rules and can accommodate individuals or many players. Healthy competition occurs as players use their knowledge and skills to correctly answer questions and gain points. Those with the highest scores are often designated as the "winners," and prizes may be awarded. Games are an effective way to incorporate visual, auditory, reading, and kinesthetic learning preferences.[12] Gaming can also be used to support competency in teamwork and collaboration as it can be completed in interprofessional settings with multidisciplinary health care providers participating.

Gamification is an innovative approach to sustain engagement and interest in learning while providing a safe and functional environment for education. Gamified education has been shown to positively influence motivation and knowledge retention.[12,14] Through active participation, continuous feedback, challenging content, and rewards, learners become immersed in the topic, resulting in increased knowledge and expansion of skills.[14]

Simulation and Role Play

Simulation is now commonplace as a strategy to educate and enhance the competence of health care professionals in a controlled setting. The standards established by the International Nursing Association for Clinical Simulation and Learning (INACSL)[15] provide evidence-based guidelines for best practice in simulation, and many nurse educators working in simulation obtain the Certified Healthcare Simulation Educator designation as part of their professional responsibility as this specialty grows.

Simulated learning is a structured process that begins with prebriefing, during which facilitators set the stage for the learning activity by reviewing learning objectives, goals of the session, participants' roles, and equipment to be used as they orient groups to the environment and explain the evaluation process.[16] It is followed by the actual simulation experience where the learner assumes a role and interacts with the focus of the learning activity. The final step is debriefing, during which the simulated scenario events are analyzed as learners are guided to reflect on their individual and group performance. During debriefing, gaps in skills are identified, and constructive feedback is provided. Simulation experiences can use low-fidelity manikins that have limited functionality or high-fidelity manikins that can be programmed to provide vital signs, pulses, cardiac rhythms, hemodynamic monitoring, and even verbal communication. The most realistic simulations use standardized patients. These individuals are carefully trained to adopt the characteristics of actual patients with specific conditions. Standardized patients realistically portray different disorders and their presentations vary based on learner roles, responses, and performance.

Simulation is widely used as a vehicle to enhance knowledge and skills appropriate to individual disciplines. In addition, the role-play aspect of simulated learning supports achievement of learning outcomes in the affective domain, which impacts learner attitudes and emotional growth and development. Adding varying degrees of complexity and enhanced technology can accommodate learning needs at all levels from novice to expert. Learning scenarios can be planned and sequential or can be unstructured and improvised; unstructured scenarios allow for spontaneous interaction between participants. Those not actively assuming a role in the simulation are considered observers and are encouraged to provide constructive feedback during the debriefing session after the scenario is completed.

Interprofessional simulations have been shown to enhance teamwork and collaboration as well as communication skills.[16,17] Too frequently, communication breakdowns occur in health care settings, putting patients at risk. Simulation with role play provides the opportunity to evaluate communication skills while providing participants with real-time feedback as they identify ways to enhance clarity. Learners see how communication styles impact information received by others and how improved communication builds confidence and trust that can positively influence teamwork and collaboration and guard against errors. With both simulation and role play, educators can allow the learning experience to be repeated after debriefing has occurred so that participants can immediately incorporate feedback they have been given. This frequently results in better outcomes, improves team interactions, and provides learners with effective strategies to use in their practice. Interprofessional team members work through the scenarios together, fostering critical thinking and emergency management skills. Learning through simulation is impactful as effective interprofessional teams are linked to better patient outcomes, fewer errors, and enhanced quality, safe care delivery.[16] Even when face-to-face simulation is not practical, interprofessional education and practice can continue through the use of electronic communication platforms.

Virtual Patient Simulation

Aspects of simulation and gaming are combined in virtual patient simulation. These interactive digital simulation platforms require licensing agreements that are purchased for institutional use and provide learners with an interactive way to experience virtual clinical scenarios without fear of harming patients. As this market grows, there is a wide selection of patient scenarios to support clinical learning that can be basic, such as respiratory assessment or complex, such as a pulseless patient or a patient experiencing an allergic reaction. Learners navigate through assessing, diagnosing, stabilizing, and teaching patients. At the conclusion of the scenarios, learners can evaluate how the selected interventions altered the outcome and impacted the delivery of quality care. Evidence-based practice, national safety standards, and social determinants of health are incorporated as the learner cares for a diverse population of patients. Users earn digital clinical experience scores as they successfully navigate the virtual patient scenario, enabling nurse educators in academia and NPD practitioners to evaluate the decision-making and clinical reasoning skills of individual learners. Debriefing after a virtual simulation supports the development of nursing knowledge and clinical judgment skills.

Immersive virtual reality simulation

Immersive virtual reality simulation is a newer and expanding form of advanced technology that provides an experiential simulation platform using a three-dimensional, computer-generated environment to replicate real-life experiences for the learner.[18,19] Learners may wear headsets, goggles, or use haptic sensors (tactic sensors) to replace environmental sensory inputs (auditory, visual, and tactile), creating a more authentic sense of interaction in real time with patients in a virtual world.

A systematic review of the effectiveness of virtual reality simulation as a learning tool in nursing education found it to be effective in improving cognitive performance and psychomotor skills.[18] This technology has been used successfully to educate health care providers about situations that are not commonly experienced but for which caregivers must be prepared for, such as high-risk deliveries, postpartum hemorrhage, and shoulder dystocia. Wu and colleagues[20] identified that past learning experiences positively affect learning outcomes related to virtual reality simulation, suggesting that nurse educators should use a variety of learning methods in meeting learning outcomes.

This newer technology has been found to be effective in nursing education regardless of the age, gender, or expertise of the learner, but barriers do exist.[18] A safe physical environment with open space should be available. Prescription glasses can make wearing headsets uncomfortable, and simulator sickness can occur. Choi and colleagues[18] reported left-handed players having difficulty with hand controls and a limited selection of available scenarios, identifying a need for more immersive virtual reality simulation scenarios to be developed for nursing education.

Technology and Nursing Skill Laboratories

Skill laboratories, like simulation, provide learning opportunities in a controlled setting where harm to patients cannot occur. The rapidly changing landscape of health care in conjunction with the continual influx of new equipment, policies, and procedures requires nurses to be technically adept. Skill laboratories afford nurses the hands-on opportunity to acquire new skills, maintain existing skills, and learn how to safely operate equipment. Learning to effectively and efficiently navigate electronic health records and electronic medical records is a critical skill that is particularly challenging to develop. Skill laboratories provide an opportunity to work within the institution's electronic health care system in a nonthreatening, unhurried environment to gather essential information required to provide safe care, while gaining confidence in one's technical skills.

Many institutions hold annual skills fairs to ensure staff maintain competency in common nursing practices as well as those skills that are infrequently used but critical when needed. Evidence-based practice, quality, and safety are reinforced with annual competency demonstrations that include indwelling urinary catheter insertions, central venous catheter dressing changes, peripheral IV insertions, application of emergency code-cart pads, and use of critical equipment, such as smart pumps and defibrillators. During the COVID-19 pandemic, much of this type of skill reinforcement was moved to online platforms for reviews, and nurse educators quickly adopted processes to take the actual hands-on skills training to the bedside and the units where nurses were working.

Just-in-Time Training

Just-in-time training is an approach that provides easily accessible education at the time it is needed. It is a type of microlearning where targeted education is provided in small learning units to review specific tasks, when "on-the-spot" training is required.[21] With just-in-time training, nurse educators or clinical experts support nurses by enabling them to practice new procedures just before performing them on patients. This process fosters learning, provides clinical support, mitigates errors, enhances patient safety, and promotes quality care delivery while improving confidence and self-efficacy.

An innovative way of providing just-in-time training is the use of quick response (QR) codes. The QR code is a small black and white image much like a barcode (**Fig. 1**). Once the image is scanned with an electronic device, such as a smartphone, the learner is directed to a specific educational destination.[22] The use of QR codes links nurses to specific websites, equipment videos, clinical updates, and new procedure demonstrations. The QR code technology is an effective tool for providing nurses with immediate access to needed information.

During the COVID-19 pandemic, just-in-time training was successfully implemented for nurses who needed to quickly learn how to prone critically ill and non-critically ill patients. It also was effectively used for nurses redeployed to understaffed high-acuity care settings as a way to provide education about new procedures or unfamiliar

Fig. 1. Vacutainer safety mechanism education QR code. (Developed by Patricia Duddy, MSN, RN, MBA, Nurse Manager NEPD Einstein Healthcare Network & Nicole Pecoraro, MSN, APRN, AGCNS-BC, CMSRN, Clinical Nurse Specialist, Einstein Healthcare Network.)

equipment. Through just-in-time training, nurses were able to demonstrate or talk through a new procedure before performing it on their patients. By doing so, nurses had more confidence, reducing the likelihood of errors. Just-in-time training is an example of nurses' adaptability to ensure quality and safety competencies are being implemented in the delivery of evidence-based patient care.

Electronic Communication Systems

NPD practitioners are charged with providing the needed education in creative and innovative ways amid the constraints of unit census expansions, inflexible nursing schedules, high patient acuity, and diverse learning needs. The traditional way of providing education in the classroom setting has become ineffective and inefficient; conventional methodologies are not responsive to the rapid changes in the work environment, often leaving staff without needed information in a timely manner. An alternative approach to education, with enhanced responsiveness and flexibility, is e-learning and electronic communication systems.[23]

Electronic communication systems have become integral to clinical practice and clinical education. A selection of an electronic communication system depends largely on the goals and learning objectives for an activity as well as available resources. Examples used for group learning include standardized learning management systems such as Blackboard or Canvas and audience response systems such as Kahoot or Poll Everywhere. For individual learning, podcasts, videos, webinars, and text messaging are useful. With the increasing number of available electronic systems, NPD practitioners have more educational tools at their disposal to promote engagement, learning, and knowledge retention.

Video conferencing platforms make it possible for more people to attend meetings and in-services, although engagement is challenged when attendees do not turn on cameras and unmute their microphones. Leading or participating in a video conference requires understanding of appropriate etiquette such as raising a hand to queue up to speak and awareness of one's visual background and on-camera activity, but they also provide engaging features such as capability to share screens, share documents, and enable real-time collaboration. Learners can be placed in small groups or work independently for a period during the video conference. Some platforms allow for audience polling, which promotes engagement and enables the NPD practitioner to assess the knowledge level of the group. Throughout the COVID-19 pandemic, hospitals successfully used video conferencing platforms to deliver essential didactic education virtually, including trauma and critical care courses and specialty certification review courses.

During the COVID-19 pandemic, video conferencing platforms provided the format for many Transition to Practice and nurse residency programs. The ability to place individuals in groups to work in breakout rooms and then later have them rejoin the larger group allowed for implementation of interactive learning strategies even though the meetings were virtual. An example of this is an exercise in which nurse residents work in small groups of four. Each group is assigned a specific evidence-based practice bundle to research, such as the central line-associated blood stream infections, catheter-associated urinary tract infection, or clostridium difficile infection bundle. Nurse residents work in their small groups, searching established health care Web sites for information about their designated evidence-based practice bundle. Each group has 25 minutes to learn the bundle well enough to teach it to others. The small groups then rejoined the larger group and provide presentations to peers. This creates an interactive learning experience where nurse residents can still work with peers on their assignments yet come into the larger group for questions and further discussion. Through this process, technology supports innovative teaching strategies that might not be used under other circumstances.

Learning management systems such as Blackboard and Canvas have long been part of academia but have recently been used in clinical practice settings to disseminate educational modules to nursing personnel. The changes due to COVID-19 created needs for social distancing and time limitations for education, prompting NPD educators to use these systems to provide didactic material before attending skills sessions. Using learning management systems in this way assisted nurses with completing online pre-work before attending face-to-face required training. In this way, in-person course time was devoted to demonstration and return demonstration of skills. Blending online learning modules with in-person skill demonstrations has been successful in maintaining the on-going and continuous education of direct care nurses.

ACCELERATION OF CHANGE IN TIME OF CRISIS

Health care professionals and organizations throughout the world were confronted with unprecedented challenges stemming from the COVID-19 pandemic. As COVID-19 emerged and worsened, the World Health Organization quickly declared it a global pandemic.[24] It became abundantly clear to health care organizations that quick operational changes were needed, and strategic plans for implementation of the changes were crucial. Technology was essential in disseminating the plan and meeting the educational needs of those providing care.

Within short windows of time, hospitals were filled beyond capacity with patients critically ill with the novel COVID-19 virus. Clinical units were transformed into additional critical care units, requiring nurses with critical care skills to care for these patients. Nurses from various specialties, such as surgical services, required immediate education to be safely redeployed to inpatient settings to take clinical assignments.[25] The crushing volume of patients continued for months, straining health care system resources and the resolve of health care providers. The unrelenting stress and physical exhaustion had profound negative effects on health care providers as they struggled to provide safe care amid dwindling supplies, insufficient staffing, emotional strain, fear of personal illness, and uncertainty about the future.

Hospitals developed command centers to provide leadership and guidance to all employees. It became essential for health care organizations to rapidly implement continuously changing safety protocols to meet regulatory requirements. In addition, in an attempt to combat the virus, the Food and Drug Administration authorized the use of multiple drugs to combat the virus, and many of the drugs were unfamiliar to health care providers. Numerous Emergency Use Authorizations were approved, requiring intense education to ensure safe administration of new medications. Educational demands were high, requiring the daily dissemination of frequent clinical changes, new guidelines, new procedures, and new restrictions.[26,27]

NPD practitioners were greatly impacted as the demand for education far exceeded the capacity of many NPD departments.[26] The need for maximal clinical support took priority over other responsibilities. As a result, many NPD practitioners were providing direct care for patients, serving on proning teams, and assisting nursing staff on clinical units. Although many education programs were suspended, nursing orientation and residency programs continued because of the need to onboard as many nurses as safely possible. Without question, all of these changes required modifications to the daily workflow of NPD teams. Despite the frenzied pace brought forward by the pandemic, quality and safe care remained a nursing priority.

NPD practitioners quickly evaluated all educational programs and in-service education requests. Prioritization strategies were developed to best meet the needs of the nursing department; immediate direct patient care training took precedence over all requests. Strict social distancing guidelines from the Centers for Disease Control and Prevention (CDC) prohibited most in-person classes from safely taking place. Technology provided a way to meet educational needs while also mitigating the spread of the COVID-19 virus. Training programs were rapidly transformed into virtual models. Video conferencing became the communication platform used for nursing orientation and all educational offerings. Breakout rooms, online simulations, videos, and webinars were used to meet learning objectives. Nursing skill laboratories required reorganization with staggered start times to limit the number of staff present in the laboratory at any one time.

Just-in-time training became the mainstay as NPD practitioners were working side by side with direct care nurses on patient care units. QR codes provided quick and easily accessed educational resources. Learning management systems were fully used as learning modules were quickly developed and widely disseminated to nursing staff. These systems proved an efficient way to quickly reach the extensive number of nurses requiring information to provide safe and effective care. The chaos of the COVID-19 pandemic created tremendous opportunities to accelerate change with innovation and creativity.

FUTURE INITIATIVES TO BRIDGE ACADEMIA AND PRACTICE

Technology in health care continues to evolve. The patient safety movement began with *To Err is Human*[28] and brought about innovative solutions that included patient care machinery with hard stops to prevent patient harm, advanced monitoring and alarm systems, and barcoding to prevent medication administration error. Patient harm was mitigated by evidence-based best practices, the initiation of checklists and timeouts, and a hypervigilance and preoccupation with error, driven by financial incentives to maintain quality and safety standards. It is hard to know the full impact that the COVID-19 pandemic will have on the health care system, but it is clear that the nursing profession met the extreme challenges with innovation and resolve and confirmed that accelerated change does not have to compromise quality.

Moving forward, partnership between academia and practice will be vital if schools of nursing are to produce an adequate number of practice-ready graduates to meet the health care needs of a traumatized society. The increased need for nurses will make it essential for academic institutions to find ways to prepare a greater number of individuals despite dwindling clinical sites, inadequate numbers of nurse faculty, and limited institutional resources. Technology will most certainly be part of that solution as classes continue to expand to online venues and virtual patient simulations provide opportunities to gain nursing knowledge and clinical experience, but considerations about different learners' level of comfort and knowledge of technology will need to be addressed. Although today's learners who are entering college are generally considered digital natives, the majority of their experience is based in mobile device applications, and it should not be assumed that these learners will naturally be proficient in educational technologies.[29]

The idea of being practice ready will include not only the ability to navigate technology in the patient care setting but will also require that bedside nurses can interpret data and effectively use dashboards to understand where improvement is possible so that practitioners can seek novel and innovative solutions to individual and systems problems. Hospital education departments will need to examine their technologies and consider how they can be used to improve care. Budgetary considerations should include academic–practice partnerships that share technology in the form of state-of-the-art simulation laboratories and immersive virtual reality systems for cost containment. The potential benefits of simulation applied to all areas of health care including mental health and primary care will need to be explored. Instructional design and Internet technologies departments will need to be expanded to manage an increased volume of support services, and planning will be required to maintain operations in the event of system failures.

The need for academic–practice partnerships was accentuated in the wake of limited student interaction with patients and the health care system due to the COVID-19 pandemic and clinical learning restrictions imposed to prevent spread. The impact of that limitation is yet to be realized. In addition, many clinical sites limit student access to computer systems to prevent breaches of privacy and systems security, hindering the learning experience.[29] Nursing programs and clinical partners will need to combine efforts to ensure that the integration of technology in nursing education is supported in the classroom as well as the clinical setting to assist the transfer of knowledge from the classroom to the patient bedside and ensure learners can navigate practice-setting technology. To prepare practice-ready professional nurses of the future, innovative and creative technology-focused teaching methods must be incorporated into curricula in both academic and practice settings as a vehicle for learning as well as a means to impact quality and safety of patient care.

SUMMARY

To promote positive patient outcomes and excellent care delivery, infusing quality and safety competencies into all educational offerings and practice expectations is essential. Despite the unprecedented obstacles stemming from the COVID-19 pandemic, NPD practitioners and nurse educators successfully harnessed educational technology to disseminate an extraordinary amount of vital information needed to provide care to a world in crisis. The agile adoption of educational technology allowed rapid access and dissemination of information that carried institutions through the uncharted waters of the pandemic and created a roadmap for mass education techniques to guide not only future disaster preparedness and crisis intervention but also application of nursing education in all arenas.

CLINICS CARE POINTS

- Nursing practice requires that nurses be competent in informatics and health care technology, and academia has responded by making it a core competency of nursing education.

- Technology in nursing education enhances learner engagement through gamification of learning, simulation, and immersive virtual learning experiences.

- Electronic communication systems make it possible to provide remote education and training to large numbers of learners with increased flexibility.

- Changing the process of education delivery will require increased investment in instructional design and information technologies support.

- Building and strengthening academic–practice partnerships is a key component in developing practice ready nurses with strong technological skills.

REFERENCES

1. Saad L. Military brass, judges among professions at new image lows. Gallup. 2021. Available at: https://news.gallup.com/poll/388649/military-brass-judges-among-professions-new-image-lows.aspx. Accessed January 13, 2022.
2. Institute of Medicine. Crossing the quality chasm: a new health system for the 21st century. Washington DC: National Academies Press; 2001. Available at: https://www.ncbi.nlm.nih.gov/books/NBK222274. Accessed October 13, 2021.
3. Cronenwett L, Sherwood G, Barnsteiner J, et al. Quality and safety education for nurses. Nurs Outlook 2007;55(3):122–31.
4. American Association of College of Nursing. The essentials: core competencies for professional nursing education. 2021. Available at: https://www.aacnnursing.org/AACN-Essentials. Accessed December 7, 2021.
5. Hopkins-Pepe L. The feasibility and effects of an orientation program framed by QSEN competencies for registered nurses. Ann Arbor, Michigan: ProQuest Dissertations Publishing; 2019 (Publication No. 13865408) [Doctoral dissertation, Widener University].
6. Sherwood G. Quality and safety education for nurses: making progress in patient safety, learning from COVID-19. Int J Nurs Sci 2021;8:249–51.
7. National Academies of Sciences, Engineering, and Medicine. The future of nursing 2020-2030: charting a path to achieve health equity. Washington, DC: The National Academies Press; 2021. https://doi.org/10.17226/25982.
8. Gronseth SL, Hutchins HM. Flexibility in formal workplace learning: technology applications for engagement through the lens of universal design for learning. Tech Trends 2021;64:211–8.
9. Pilcher J, Graebe J. Strategies to promote learning and engage participants. J Contin Educ Nurs 2018;49(5):197–9.
10. Chicca J, Shellenbarger T. Generation Z: approaches and teaching-learning practices for nursing professional development practitioners. J Nurses Prof Dev 2018;34(5):250–6.

11. Weinschreider J, Sabourin KM, Smith CM. Preparing nurse leaders in nursing professional development: educational technology resources. J Nurses Prof Dev 2019;35(5):281–5.
12. Woolwine S, Romp CR, Jackson B. Game on: evaluating the impact of gamification in nursing orientation on motivation and knowledge retention. J Nurses Prof Dev 2019;35(5):255–60. https://doi.org/10.1097/NND.0000000000000570.
13. Fijacko N, Gosak L, Debeljak N, et al. Gamification in nursing: a literature review. Obzornik Zdravstvene Nege 2020;54(2):133–52.
14. Murad S. Brain involvement in the use of games in nursing education. J Nurs Educ Pract 2017;7(6):90–4.
15. International Nursing Association for Clinical Simulation and Learning (INACSL). Healthcare Simulation Standards of Best Practice. 2021. Available at: https://www.inacsl.org/healthcare-simulation-standards. Accessed December 30, 2021.
16. Poore J, Cooper D. Interprofessional simulation: from the classroom to clinical practice. Annu Rev Nurs Res 2020;39(1):105–25.
17. Liaw SY, Choo T, Wu LT, et al. Wow, woo, win—healthcare students' and facilitators' experiences of interprofessional simulation in three-dimensional world: a qualitative evaluation study. Nurse Educ Today 2021;105:1–6.
18. Choi J, Thompson E, Choi J, et al. Effectiveness of immersive virtual reality in nursing education. Nurse Educ 2021. https://doi.org/10.1097/NNE.0000000000000117.
19. Zackoff M, Lin L, Israel K, et al. The future of onboarding: implementation of immersive virtual reality for nursing clinical assessment training. J Nurses Prof Dev 2020;36(4):235–40.
20. Wu SH, Huang CC, Huang SS, et al. Effect of virtual reality training to decreases rates of needle stick/sharp injuries in new-coming medical and nursing interns in Taiwan. J Educ Eval Health Prof 2020;17:1.
21. Patel S, Hartung B, Nagra R, et al. Expedited cross-training: an approach to help mitigate nurse staffing shortages. Nurses Prof Dev 2021;37(6):E20–6.
22. Bradley K. Just-in-time learning and QR codes: a must-have tool for nursing professional development specialists. J Contin Educ Nurs 2020;51(7):302–3.
23. White M, Shellenbarger T. Harnessing the power of learning management systems: an E-learning approach for professional development. J Nurses Prof Dev 2017;33(3):138–41.
24. Dale-Tam J, Thompson K. Nursing orientation during the COVID-19 pandemic. J Nurses Prof Dev 2021;37(4):216–9.
25. Hermann M, Blizzard T, Carve R, et al. Implementing a nursing skills practice laboratory using social distancing during the COVID-19 pandemic. J Nurses Prof Dev 2021;37(4):206–10.
26. Fox N, Richter S. The nursing professional development practitioner during a pandemic: achieving the hat trick. J Nurses Prof Dev 2021;37(3):E5–9.
27. Sites C, Templin C. When crisis strikes, handle with care. J Nurses Prof Dev 2021;37(3):151–3. https://doi.org/10.1097/NND.0000000000000707.
28. Kohn LT, Corrigan JM, Donaldson MS, editors. To err is human: building a safer health system. Washington DC: National Academies Press; 2000. Available at: https://www.nap.edu/read/9728/chapter/1. Accessed November 14, 2021.
29. Smart D, Ross K, Carolio S, et al. Contextualizing instructional technology to the demands of nursing education. Comput Inform Nurs 2020;23(1):18–27.

Best Practices for Facilitating the Mentoring Experience for Nursing Students of Color

Yolanda M. Nelson, EdD, MSN-Ed, RN-BC

KEYWORDS

- Academic success • Cultural diversity • e-mentoring • Ethnic and racial minorities
- Mentors • Minority groups • Nursing education • Social inclusion

KEY POINTS

- Providing a mentoring environment that is caring, supportive, and values all races and ethnic backgrounds promotes engagement and increases retention rates of nursing students of color.
- Effective mentorship requires commitment, time, support, and open lines of communication from both the mentor and mentee.
- Mentorship can support the recruitment and retention of students of color and can contribute to a culturally diverse workforce representative of the population.
- Key elements in the development of a successful mentorship program include partnering with stakeholders, training collaborators to perform their roles effectively, and clearly communicating goals to align expectations and keep mentees and mentors informed.

INTRODUCTION

Nursing is lacking in diversity. According to a 2017 survey, the majority of registered nurses (RNs) are White/Caucasian (80.8%), 7.5% are Asian, 6.2% are African American, 5.3% are Hispanic, and less than 1% are American Indian/Alaskan Native or Native Hawaiian/Pacific Islander.[1] The nursing profession does not mirror the diversity of the population it serves despite numerous efforts to increase diversity among nurses. Efforts to expand diversity in nursing are critical because nursing diversity plays a significant role in an individual's perceptions of their health needs, and it affects their response to health care.[2] Literature confirms that minority nurses are valuable contributors to the provision of health care services in this country as well as leaders in the development of models of care designed to address the unique needs of minority populations.[1]

School of Nursing and Health Sciences, Trenton Hall, 2000 Pennington Road, Ewing, NJ 08628, USA
E-mail address: nelsony1@tcnj.edu

Nurs Clin N Am 57 (2022) 563–573
https://doi.org/10.1016/j.cnur.2022.06.006
0029-6465/22/© 2022 Elsevier Inc. All rights reserved.

To improve diversity in the nursing profession, many colleges and universities are making efforts to increase and retain students of color so that RNs as a group begin to reflect the population they serve presently and will serve in the future. The literature describes the impact of retention strategies geared toward supporting student progression and successful licensure to practice.[3-7] One driving force supporting student success and contributing to diversity within the nursing profession is mentorship. Mentorship can offer a means to enhance workforce performance and engagement, promote learning opportunities, and encourage multidisciplinary collaboration.[8] Increasing diversity in schools of nursing is key to increasing diversity in the nursing workforce.[9]

To better understand and improve current mentoring practices, it is essential to examine what is—and what is not—currently working in existing mentorship programs and models and to explore areas that have not been tapped for mentoring. The following sections provide a review of current best practices for mentoring nursing students of color and recommendations to move these practices forward.

Definition of Terms

In the context of this article, key terms are defined as follows:

Students of color: students who identify as Black or African American, Latina or Latino, Asian, Native American, or multiple of the above-mentioned racial identities.

Mentoring: refers to providing support, encouragement, advice, and role modeling, and can be short-term or long-term.

Mentoring relationship: refers to a professional, meaningful relationship between nurses and nursing students in the classroom, through their clinical work and in other areas of their training and personal growth.

E-mentoring (digital): a computer-mediated, mutually beneficial relationship between a mentor and a mentee that provides learning, advising, encouraging, promoting, and role modeling that differs from face-to-face mentoring.

Mentorship

The process of becoming a nurse can be a difficult and stressful journey that includes ups, downs, lack of self-confidence, challenges, barriers, and rewards. The difficulties during the journey of being a college student can, at times, lead to uncertainty and lack of confidence and may deter students from completing nursing school. Research indicates that the attrition rate can be as high as 85% for minority nursing students.[10] Challenges and barriers to success may include lack of time management skills, poor academic preparation, language barriers, financial barriers, a sense of not fitting in, and a highly competitive environment. Considering the challenges, struggles, and barriers that they may face, what tools should be provided for nursing students of color? Evidence in the literature validates mentorship as an effective tool to increase persistence and success among nursing students of color.

The concept of a mentor dates back thousands of years to a character in Homer's poem, "The Odyssey." Odysseus hired Mentor, a wise and trusted advisor who assumed many roles throughout the narrative to care for and educate his son, Telemachus.[11] Today, a mentor is viewed as a role model, advisor, sharer of knowledge, and an active part of a support system. Mentorship models have been used in schools of nursing since as far back as the 1980s. Currently, numerous nursing schools actively use mentorship models and programs to support and provide resources to students of color so that they may graduate successfully and become leaders in the profession of nursing.

MENTORSHIP AND ITS SIGNIFICANCE

Compared with other students, nursing students of ethnic minority backgrounds have lower graduation rates, which have been attributed to lack of academic preparation, social support, and financial resources.[12] Mentorship before nursing school is an important factor in the success of ethnic minority students. Payton and colleagues[12] found that mentorship aided African American nursing students in four main areas: test-taking skills, isolation and loneliness, diversity, and support.

The value of mentorship in helping nursing students from minority groups succeed in nursing school is far greater in comparison to other efforts to support them. Mentoring is a leading method to help socialize students to the profession of nursing.[5] Mentoring emerges through having a knowledgeable nurse leader (mentor) guide the student (mentee) as they progress through nursing school. Several studies have reported mentorship as being a vital influence in the persistence of African American students.[13,14] Mentorship is powerful, provides personal development, and is an inspirational tool. It involves mutual trust and respect and provides an effective way of assisting the progression of others. A mentor offers advice, provides guidance, creates open lines of communication, shares life experiences, provides helpful feedback, and enriches the mentoring relationship. When mentoring is executed correctly, the experience tends to be holistic, touching the mind and the heart. Mentoring can be provided in an informal (unstructured) or formal (structured) manner. Developing a mentoring relationship can assist a student to understand their full potential, enhance their self-esteem, act as a confidence booster, and serve as a networking opportunity. Key aspects of a mentoring relationship include collaboration, commitment, active participation, communication, role modeling, engagement, and a caring environment. The purpose of this article is to provide guidelines for establishing effective mentorship programs by (1) reviewing the literature regarding the best practices for mentoring nursing students of color, and (2) exploring the role of e-mentoring (digital mentoring) in nursing education.

REVIEW OF THE LITERATURE

Two questions guided a review of the literature: (1) What does the literature say about the best practices of mentoring students of color? and (2) How does technology play a role in facilitating the mentoring experience? Literature published since 2001 on mentoring opportunities for nursing students of color was selected from multiple databases including the Cumulative Index to Nursing and Allied Health (CINAHL), PubMed, and Education Resources Information Center (ERIC). Searches were conducted using a variety of terms including students of color, mentoring, nursing students, minority, nursing, mentorship programs, and health care profession. Inclusion and exclusion criteria and search terms are presented in **Table 1**.

An initial review of the abstracts was followed by a more in-depth review of the full-text articles. A critical analysis based on the main concepts of the literature review led to the identification of the themes presented in **Table 2**.

FINDINGS

It is important to begin an identification of best practices by examining the characteristics and outcomes of mentorship programs that have been offered to nursing students of color. Many universities now sponsor formalized mentoring relationships with the goal of improving educational and career opportunities for women, ethnic minorities, and returning older students; all of whom are less likely to have a formal

Table 1
Inclusion criteria and exclusion criteria, created by the author

Inclusion Criteria	
Criterion 1: Time duration	Articles within the last 20 years
Criterion 2: Keywords	Mentoring, nursing, students of color, diverse, digital mentoring, best practices, mentoring models, and programs
Criterion 3: Publication	Peer review process
Criterion 4: Content	Language in English
Criterion 5: Research	Empirical research
Criterion 6: E-Mentoring	Mentorship programs using e-mentoring (digital)
Criterion 7: Participants	Nurses and nursing students
Exclusion Criteria	
Criterion 1: Relation	Not related to mentoring, e-mentoring, and mentorship programs for students of color
Criterion 2: Peer review	Articles did not undergo a peer review process
Criterion 3: Research	Articles did not include a research method
Criterion 4: Mentorship	Mentorship program that serviced the general population
Criterion 5: Content	Language other than English
Criterion 6: Participants	Other health professionals (besides nursing)

mentor.[15] In a study by Mills and Wisneski,[16] students reported that they believed a mentor would assist them to be more successful in their nursing program. Several studies reported mentorship as being a vital influence in the persistence of African American students.[13,14] The findings related to the importance of mentorship and

Table 2
Best practices of mentoring nursing students of color

Factors	Characteristics
Communication	Active listening
	Goal setting
	Formal/informal
	Willingness to share knowledge
	Open, honest feedback
	Sharing experiences
	Online platform communication
	Approachability
	Effective interpersonal skills
Commitment	Commitment of time
	Setting boundaries
	Develop a mentor/mentee contract
	Take responsibility
	Accountability
	Effective mentorship
Training	Keys to being a mentor
	Cultural competency
	Ongoing education
	Rapport
Right fit	Appropriate
	Skills and goals
	Engagement

advisement as a means of social and academic advancement confirm the work of Davis-Dick[14] who offered five recommendations for developing a strong and effective mentor–mentee relationship: dedication, honesty and trust, mutual respect, a positive and caring attitude, and appreciation.

Analysis of the literature related to mentorship programs for nursing students of color revealed several successful practices that helped increase diversity within the nursing workforce. Those best practices identified within the mentorship programs encompass the following four themes: communication, dedication to the process, mentor training/education, and the right fit.

Theme 1: The Art of Communication

Communication. Effective communication, both verbal and nonverbal, is necessary when developing a solid and trusting mentoring relationship. Mentorship allows the mentor–mentee to share knowledge of their life and personal experiences, collaborate, and listen to one another's viewpoint. This may include the mentor sharing of wisdom on test-taking skills, how to study, and note taking. Communication plays a significant role in the satisfaction on the part of both the mentor and mentee.[17] Suggestions to support effective communication between the mentor and mentee include discussing clear expectations and developing goals that are specific, measurable, achievable, relevant, and time-bound (SMART goals). Setting SMART goals provides structure for the mentoring process.[18] Cypress[19] concluded that a fruitful mentor–mentee relationship includes having good communication that is open and thoughtful, allowing the mentor and mentee to listen to one another. Lee and colleagues[20] described the importance of maintaining effective communication as the key to any mentor–mentee relationship with no exceptions. It is important for both the mentor and mentee to understand their own communication styles and take time to practice communication skills.[20]

Theme 2: Dedication to the Process

Commitment. Before developing a mentoring relationship, both the mentor and mentee must understand that such a relationship involves dedication, enthusiasm, and intentionality in the process. A mentor–mentee relationship is one that involves mutual respect, time, and dedication. Vance,[21] an innovator in nursing mentorship research, states that a commitment and passion for a professional career and a yearning to excel and succeed are essential in a mentoring relationship. For an effective mentoring relationship to occur, one must be committed to developing the mentoring bond.[7]

Theme 3: Mentor Training and Education

Training and education. There are times when a mentor may not understand what a mentoring relationship involves. Training can assist mentors in understanding various cultures, ways to communicate, and how to sustain a mentoring relationship. Findings from a qualitative study identified the importance of providing mentors with support to carry out their role.[7] An important component of best practices in mentorship programs is providing culturally competent training to mentors.[5] Nelson and colleagues[17] reported that training on mentor–mentee relationships is mandatory for mentors in their "Moving Forward Together" mentorship program, which aims to meet the needs of African American nursing students. Along with information on mentor–mentee relationships, workshops should be offered to mentors and mentees to assist in answering questions, networking, and developing strong bonds between the mentor and mentee.[17] Rhodes[22] recommends providing more than 6 hours of training to mentors that includes post-match training (after mentors are matched with their mentees).

Information presented during training may include building rapport with the mentee, learning how to set goals, and teaching the value of having a presence.

Theme 4: The Right Fit

Mentor–Mentee match. Nickitas[6] asserted that an appropriate fit is important for creating a successful mentor–mentee relationship; therefore, matching the right mentor to the right mentee is the fourth-best practice theme. Nelson and colleagues[17] also identified matching as an important best practice in creating the mentoring relationship. A mentor and mentee should share some commonality in goals, skills, similar area of focus, cultural background, and accomplishments.

Rapport. It is essential to understand that after one finds the "right fit," the mentor and mentee must also develop rapport with each other. Finding opportunities to build and develop personal connections between mentors and mentees is central to initiating and preserving a mentoring relationship.[23]

TECHNOLOGY: E-MENTORING (DIGITAL) MODELS

In addition to the four themes related to mentorship programs for nursing students of color, many of the studies addressed the role of technology in mentoring. Technology use has increased over the past 5–10 years and has become an important facilitator in building a mentoring relationship by making significant and innovative contributions to the field of mentorship and mentoring models. During the COVID-19 pandemic, communication had to shift from face-to-face contact to a digital environment. Mentors and mentees have used various digital and virtual platforms that include audio and visual elements ranging from widely familiar technology such as texting and telephone calls to more sophisticated virtual platforms such as Zoom, FaceTime, and Microsoft Teams. Many faculty and students learned through this experience that digital applications offer an effective way for mentors and mentees to communicate. E-mentoring can be described as "a computer-mediated, mutually beneficial relationship between a mentor and a mentee which provides learning, advising, encouraging, promoting, and modeling different than face-to-face mentoring."[24(p.212)] E-mentoring is a somewhat new approach to mentoring in nursing education and provides cost-effective experiences and learning opportunities in a flexible environment.[25] Digital mentoring may emerge as an important way to significantly increase diversity within the profession of nursing. In the next 5–10 years, as virtual reality becomes a more prominent medium for simulation, it may also provide a more sophisticated medium for digital mentoring.[26]

A limited number of peer-reviewed articles have described e-mentoring (digital) models. In an analysis of an e-mentoring program, Mollica and Mitchell[27] concluded that online mentorship programs can offer the support that undergraduate nursing students need. They found that e-mentoring reduced anxiety, was convenient for both the mentor and mentee, and increased student confidence and interaction. Welch[28] noted that the digital mentoring environment is flexible and convenient for the mentors and mentees. Gregg and colleagues[29] concluded that as more students use online learning for instruction, virtual student support services have the potential to improve student engagement and retention.

Benefits and Pitfalls of E-Mentoring

Few articles have addressed the challenges and benefits of e-mentoring. Although e-mentoring is relatively new, there are many benefits to this approach to mentoring.[27–29] E-mentoring allows individuals to develop a purposeful relationship with the assistance of technology that might not otherwise be practical or possible. More-over, e-mentoring offers the potential to increase the mentor pool and make it more diverse as mentors can be in more distant locations. Mentees may feel less intimi-dated and isolated by interacting with their mentor in a digital environment. Potential mentors may find that they have more time to engage with their mentees by using the e-mentoring model. Communicating electronically also helps mentees build their on-line communication abilities. E-mentoring can assist in closing generational gaps be-tween nurses, students, and faculty, and it can allow learning to emerge in both directions between mentors and mentees.[30] Mentees can engage with nurse leaders and build relationships with diverse individuals across the world. Lastly, the digital mentoring experience supports the creation of a comfortable environment for the mentor and mentee.

There are also some challenges that require attention when considering e-mentor-ing. Available technology support and resources are needed, especially as technology evolves and advances in complexity. Another concern is digital communication in a virtual environment where the mentor or mentee may not readily pick up on verbal cues such as body language. Moreover, digital and virtual environments can pose some risks to privacy and confidentiality.

LIMITATIONS

Although a thorough review of the literature was conducted, there is a possibility that articles and programs were missed. When considering e-mentoring, there is an insuf-ficient number of studies evaluating the effectiveness of technology-driven mentoring for nursing students of color. It is important to note that the findings in this article reflect current practices in mentoring nursing students of color at the time the literature review was conducted.

FUTURE DIRECTIONS

Further exploration and development of best practices in mentoring nursing students of color should include the following:

- Innovative and evidence-based development of future mentoring strategies,
- Further research regarding the process of e-mentoring (digital mentoring),
- Development of collaborations with nursing organizations that support under-graduate nursing students of color,
- Provision of training in cultural competence to nurse faculty, mentors, and staff,
- More funding of opportunities to enhance current and future mentorship pro-grams and models,
- Additional research regarding the ethical issues and difficulties of mentorship,
- Research and dissemination related to key components of mentorship programs and mentoring models,
- Efforts to address the high attrition rates of nursing students of color.

Recommendations for future directions and relevant resources for implementing these recommendations are presented in **Table 3**.

SUGGESTIONS FOR GETTING STARTED

When considering future directions, the first step is to review the current literature regarding programs that are geared toward meeting the needs of nursing students of color. Two questions that should be considered are as follows: (1) *What does the*

Table 3 Recommendations for future directions	
Recommendations	**Resources**
Development of mentoring strategies	• Robert Wood Johnson Foundation—New Careers in Nursing Mentor Program Toolkit[31]
Nursing organizations for development of collaborations	• American Nurses Association—Collaborative Activity[32] • American Association of Colleges of Nursing[33] • National League for Nursing[34] • National Black Nurses Association[35]
Cultural competency training	• Health workforce cultural competency interventions[36]
Funding sources	• National League for Nursing[34] • Health Resources and Services Administration (HRSA)[37]

current evidence state about the facilitation of a mentor–mentee relationship? and (2) *What does the literature say about effective mentoring and engagement strategies?* Once you have a foundation in the literature, it is essential to review exemplary mentorship programs and identify the criteria that characterize your criteria for a successful mentorship program. Those criteria may include measures of graduation rates, NCLEX pass rates, and retention of mentors and mentees. Also consider characteristics of mentorship programs that would fit your ideal model, including resources, involvement of stakeholders, mentoring strategies, theoretical frameworks, types of mentorship programs (traditional, group, peer, or e-mentoring), collaborative partners (if any), and trainings. It is important to note that as you begin the development of a mentorship program or a mentoring relationship, it is vital to have the support of your organization. An environment that supports a culture of mentorship is central to the sustainability of any mentorship program.

Collaborations with other organizations, such as another college, university, or health care organization, can be beneficial for both parties in the collaboration. Before building a collaborative relationship, consider the following factors:

1. *Partnering* with a local hospital affiliate, health care organization, or another university or college. Additional collaborative partners may include local high schools and middle schools.
2. *Involving stakeholders*, such as hospital administrators, nurses, students, nursing faculty, college administrators, and professional development leaders. Each stakeholder should play a pivotal function in the mentorship program, and their roles should clearly be defined.
3. *Training collaborators*, so that everyone understands their role and anticipated contributions to the mentorship program.
4. *Communicating clearly* with everyone involved, and setting specified meeting times to keep all collaborative partners informed and updated.

SUMMARY

To meet the existing and future health care needs of people from minority populations and provide culturally competent care, endeavors are needed to increase nurses' educational attainment among minority populations. Commitment to improving diversity in nursing requires creative efforts in discovering and enhancing approaches to mentorship. An atmosphere that promotes mentorship is crucial for faculty, nurses, and students of color to feel acknowledged, confident, and a sense of belonging at their institutions. Mentoring is a meaningful educational strategy that needs further investigation and integration into programs that include diverse student populations. It provides a way to develop and maintain an inclusive environment essential for the recruitment and retention of diverse students. Traditional mentoring approaches continue to be at the forefront of nursing education practice, but with the advancement of technology, options for e-mentoring continue to expand and play an important role in nursing education and advancement of diversity within the nursing profession. In the long run, effective mentorship programs will support and strengthen the nursing workforce, lay the groundwork for lifelong professional relationships, create strong nurse leaders, and contribute to better patient care and outcomes.

CLINICS CARE POINTS

- Key aspects of a mentoring relationship include collaboration, commitment, active participation, communication, role modeling, engagement, and a caring environment.
- Best mentoring practices that support nursing student success and increase diversity in the nursing workforce include communication, dedication to the process, mentor training and education, and a good mentor–mentee fit.
- Training for mentors and mentees is essential and should include mentor–mentee roles and relationships, communication, goal setting, networking, and use of technology to facilitate and sustain the mentoring relationship.
- E-mentoring facilitates mentorship relationships by mitigating challenges posed by distance and busy schedules, and further advances in technology have the potential to extend the power of digital modes of mentorship.
- Mentorship programs for nursing students of color can be strengthened through collaborations with external partners.

DISCLOSURE

"The author has nothing to disclose."

REFERENCES

1. American Association of Colleges of Nursing. Enhancing diversity in the nursing workforce. 2019. Available at: https://www.aacnnursing.org/news-information/fact-sheets/enhancing-diversity. Accessed September 10, 2021.
2. Nair L, Oluwaseun AA. Cultural competence and ethnic diversity in healthcare. Plast Reconstr Surg Glob Open 2019;7(5):e2219.
3. Sutherland JA, Hamilton MJ, Goodman N. J. Affirming at-risk minorities for success (ARMS): retention, graduation, and success on the NCLEX-RN. Nurse Educ 2007;46(8):347–53.
4. Crooks N. Mentoring as the key to minority success in nursing education. ABNF J 2013;24(2):47–50.
5. Metcalfe SE. Creative and innovative program for improving diverse students in education. Int Arch Nurse Health Care 2015. https://doi.org/10.23937/2469-5823/150015.
6. Nickitas DM. Mentorship in nursing. Nurs Econ 2014;32:2.

7. Myall M, Jones TL, Work BB, et al. Mentorship in contemporary practice: the experiences of nursing students and practice mentors. J Clin Nurs 2008. https://doi.org/10.1111/J.1365-2702.2007.02233.

8. Burgess A, Diggele CV, Mellis C. Mentorship in the health professions: a review. Clin Teach 2018. https://doi.org/10.1111/tct.12756.

9. Sullivan Commission on Diversity in the Healthcare Workforce. Missing persons: minorities in the health professions. 2014. Available at: http://www.aacn.nche.edu/media-relations/SullivanReport.pdf. Accessed September 10, 2021.

10. Gilchrist KL, Rector C. Can you keep them? Strategies to attract and retain nursing students from diverse populations: Best practices in nursing education. J Transcult Nurs 2007;18:277–85.

11. Dunk G.G. and Craft A., The road to Ithaca: a mentee's and mentor's journey, Teacher Development, 8, 2007, 277–295.

12. Payton TD, Howe LA, Timmons SM, et al. African American nursing students' perceptions about mentoring. Nurse Educ Perspect 2013;34(3):173–7. https://doi.org/10.5480/1536-5026-34.3.173.

13. Veal JL, Bull MJ, Miller JF. A framework of academic persistence and success for ethnically diverse graduate nursing students. Nurse Educ Perspect 2012;33(5):322–7.

14. Davis-Dick LR. Mentoring African American nursing students: a holistic approach. 2008. Available at: http://www.minoritynurse.com/article/mentoring-African American-nursing-students-holistic-approach. Accessed August 2, 2019.

15. Santos SJ, Reigadas ET. Understanding the student-faculty mentoring process: its effects on at-risk university students. J Coll Student Retention Res Theor Pract 2004;6(3):337–57.

16. Mills-Wisneski S. Minority students' perceptions concerning the presence of minority faculty: inquiry and discussion. J Multicultural Nurs Health 2005;11(2):49–55.

17. Nelson YM, Mohan A, Chahir Y. The mentoring experience: perceptions of African American nurse leaders and student mentees. J Nurse Educ 2021;60(1):25–8.

18. American Psychological Association. Introduction to Mentoring: A Guide for Mentors and Mentees. 2017. Available at: http://www.apa.org/education/grad/mentoring.aspx. Accessed September 10, 2021.

19. Cypress, BS. Fostering effective mentoring relationships in qualitative research educational dimension. doi: 10.1097/DCC.0000000000000444.

20. Lee SP, McGee R, Branchaw J. Mentoring up": learning to manage your mentoring relationships. Syracuse (NY): The Graduate School Press of Syracuse University; 2015.

21. Vance C, Nickitas DM. Mentorship in nursing: an interview with connie vance. Nurs Econ 2014;32(2):65–9.

22. Rhodes JE. A model of youth mentoring. In: Dubois DL, Karcher MJ, editors. Handbook of youth mentoring. Ltd: Sage Publications; 2005. p. 30–43.

23. Davey ZD, Jackson D. The value of nurse mentoring relationships: Lessons learnt from a work-based resilience enhancement programme for nurses working in the forensic setting. Int J Ment Health Nurs 2020. https://doi.org/10.1111/inm.12739.

24. Bierema LL, Merriam SB. E-mentoring: Using computer mediated communication to enhance the mentoring process. Innovative Higher Educ 2002;26(3):211–27.

25. Clement SA, Welch S. Virtual mentoring in nursing education: a scoping review of the literature. J Nurse Educ Pract 2017. https://doi.org/10.5430/jnep.v8n3p137.

26. Williams PW, Klimberg V, Perez A. Tele-education assisted mentorship in surgery (TEAMS). J Surg Oncol 2021. https://doi.org/10.1002/jso.26495.

27. Mollica M, Mitchell A. Increasing retention and student satisfaction utilizing an on-line peer mentoring program: preliminary results. Social Behav Sci 2013;106(1): 1455–61.
28. Welch MV. Evaluation of a national e-mentoring program for ethnically diverse student nurse-midwives and student midwives. 2017. Available at: https://doiorg. ezproxy.tcnj.edu/10.1111/jmwh.12547. Accessed September 10, 2021.
29. Gregg N, Galyardt A, Wolfe G, et al. Virtual mentoring and persistence in STEM for students with disabilities. Career Develop Transit Exceptional Individuals 2016;40(4). https://doi.org/10.1177/2165143416651717.
30. Clement S. The use of virtual mentoring in nursing education. Online J Nurs Inform Online J Nurs Inform 2014;18(2):1–3.
31. Robert Wood Johnson Foundation. New Careers in Nursing- Mentor Program Toolkit. Available at: http://www.newcareersinnursing.org/resources/mentoring-toolkit-and-handbook.html. Accessed January 30, 2022.
32. American Nurses Association. Collaborative Activity. Available at. https://www. nursingworld.org/practice-policy/health-policy/health-system-reform/quality/ collaborative-activity/. Accessed January 30, 2022.
33. American Association of College of Nursing. Available at. https://www. aacnnursing.org/. Accessed February 23, 2022.
34. National League for Nursing. Available at. https://www.nln.org/. Accessed February 23, 2022.
35. National Black Nurses Association. Available at. https://www.nbna.org/. Access February 23, 2022.
36. Jongen C, McCalman J, Brainbridge R. Health workforce cultural competency interventions: a systematic scoping review. BMC Health Serv Res 2018;18:232.
37. Health Resources and Services Administration. Available at. https://www.hrsa. gov/. Accessed February 23, 2022.

Frameworks and Technology for Triangulation of Feedback to Support Learning

Joni Tornwall, PhD, RN[a],*, Sarah Rusnak, MS, RD, LD[b]

KEYWORDS

- Academic performance • Competency-based education • Educational assessment
- Educational technology • Metacognition • Peer review • Professional competence
- Self-assessment

KEY POINTS

- Traditional forms of summative assessment provide for formal evaluation of learning, but they also tend to discourage students from engaging with feedback in ways that support performance improvement.
- Formative feedback and assessment processes contribute to learner engagement and competency achievement.
- Triangulation of feedback from instructors, peers, and self-reflection provides opportunities for learning and development of professional maturity.
- Emphasis on peer review processes in the classroom develops key metacognitive skills for future nursing practice and lifelong learning.
- Skillful integration of learning technologies to support assessment for learning (as well as assessment of learning) supports student engagement in competency achievement.

Traditional approaches to assessment and feedback in health care education tend to focus on high-stakes evaluation at the end of an instructional unit and result in a pass-or-fail judgment of performance. This type of assessment, referred to by educators as *summative assessment*, is a necessary part of the educational process because it allows for evaluation of student achievement of competencies on a graded scale. Although summative assessments provide the opportunity to formally evaluate student performance, they typically do not foster opportunities to provide supportive feedback intended to promote growth.[1] In contrast to summative assessment, *formative assessment* tends to focus on low-stakes learning opportunities that generate feedback aimed at improvement in student performance.[2] Even when students receive high-quality

[a] The Ohio State University College of Nursing, 1585 Neil Avenue, Columbus, OH 43210, USA;
[b] School of Health and Rehabilitation Sciences, The Ohio State University College of Medicine, 453 West 10th Avenue, Columbus, OH 43210, USA
* Corresponding author.
E-mail address: tornwall.2@osu.edu

Nurs Clin N Am 57 (2022) 575–588
https://doi.org/10.1016/j.cnur.2022.06.007
0029-6465/22/© 2022 Elsevier Inc. All rights reserved.

feedback after a summative assessment of their learning, they may not be in an ideal frame of mind to receive the feedback and use it to improve.[1] They still need to know how they performed on the summative assessment and the rationale for the score they received, but the best opportunities for learning and growth come from formative assessment—that is, assessment *for* learning rather than assessment *of* learning.[3]

An assessment culture of learning can be cultivated in the classroom by supporting a self-regulated, metacognitive approach to instruction and encouraging achievement by instilling a desire for mastery of competencies rather than proof of performance through good grades. When assessments are designed as an open dialogue within a classroom culture of learning, students have an opportunity to consider their strengths and weaknesses in a safe environment and reflect on actions needed to improve performance.[4] Assessments designed for learning rather than judgment have an integrated feedback component based on three key types of feedback information: instructor feedback, peer feedback, and self-reflection. Nurse educators can integrate these three types of feedback into formative assessments by using frameworks focused on self-regulated learning and learning technologies that are aligned well with assessment activities.

Frameworks

By helping students develop skills in metacognitive processing of feedback and self-reflection, instructors foster student engagement in lifelong learning and prepare nurses for the workplace. Traditionally, structured academic settings tend to build a performance environment in which students feel a need to prove they are competent through grades, scores, or marks. In contrast, an instructor who fosters a student's ability to self-regulate their learning through metacognition and self-reflection encourages a drive to master competencies and continuously improve performance.[5] Students who have not yet developed skills in metacognition and self-reflection tend to look only for positive feedback from assessment events and shield themselves from constructive or critical feedback.

By using frameworks from the American Association of College of Nursing (AACN) and scholars in higher education assessment, nurse educators can guide students to become feedback seekers who welcome input from colleagues and peers and know how to reflect and act on the feedback information. Helping students find ways to extract value from all feedback they receive prepares them for dynamic workplace environments where they will certainly encounter feedback that challenges their resilience and development as a health care professional.[3,6]

Competencies in Nursing and Leadership

The *AACN Core Competencies for Professional Nursing Education* (also called the AACN Essentials) outlines curricular content and core competencies expected of graduates from nursing programs.[7] The AACN supports competency-based education for nurses, which is defined as "a system of instruction, assessment, feedback, self-reflection, and academic reporting that is based on students showing that they have learned the knowledge, attitudes, motivations, self-perceptions, and skills expected of them as they progress through their education."[8] Competency-based assessments align well with the approach to feedback described in this article in that they are authentic and based on real performance (as opposed to multiple-choice examinations, for example); include external perspectives and self-assessment; and are progressive, iterative, and linked over time.[8]

The AACN Essentials form a competency-based framework that includes competency domains of Professionalism (accountability and collaborative disposition reflecting the values of nursing) and Personal, Professional, and Leadership Development (participation in activities and self-reflection leading to resilience, lifelong learning, and acquisition of expertise). **Table 1** lists specific AACN competencies and sub-competencies related to skills in giving and receiving feedback that are key to ensuring quality, safety, and continuous improvement in patient care, accountability to nursing professional standards, flexibility and professional maturity in nurses, and excellent communication among team members.[7]

Table 1
Focal competencies from AACN essentials and alignment with EAT framework dimensions

AACN Competencies and Sub-competencies[7]	EAT Framework (Instructor) Practice Areas (Adapted for Nursing education)[11]	EAT Framework Questions for Student Self-Reflection (Adapted for Nursing education)[12]
9.3 Demonstrate accountability to the individual, society, and the profession.		
9.3 h Engage in peer evaluation.	AF3: Prepare students to give and receive peer feedback	AF3: Have I prepared to participate in feedback conversations and provide supportive feedback to peers?
9.3 L Foster a practice environment that promotes accountability for care outcomes.	AL1: Clarify what constitutes "good" performance on an assessment AL4: Define nursing- and specialty-specific standards of practice and use them as benchmarks in assessment	AL1: What standards or competencies am I aiming to meet? AL4: Am I aware of the main ways of working and thinking in nursing?
10.2 Demonstrate a spirit of inquiry that fosters flexibility and professional maturity.		
10.2a Engage in guided and spontaneous reflection of one's practice.	AL3: Clarify instructor, student, and peer roles in assessment and feedback	AL3: Do I know what feedback should look like, what support is available, and what my role is in feedback?
10.2 b Integrate comprehensive feedback to improve performance.	AL2: Align how assessment elements fit together AD2: Promote meaningful, focused, real-world assessments	AL2: Do I understand how different assessment elements fit together across modules and why I am being assessed in the way I am?
10.2 h Mentor others in the development of their professional growth and accountability.	AD4: Ensure ongoing evaluation through iterative cycles of feedback	AD4: Am I giving useful feedback to peers to enhance their learning and to course faculty to improve the assessment process?
10.2i Foster activities that support a culture of lifelong learning.	AF1: Provide accessible feedback focused on improvement AF2. Provide early opportunities for feedback aligned with summative assessments	AF1: Do I know how to use the feedback I receive to meet standards and competencies and close gaps in my performance?

(continued on next page)

Table 1
(continued)

AACN Competencies and Sub-competencies[7]	EAT Framework (Instructor) Practice Areas (Adapted for Nursing education)[11]	EAT Framework Questions for Student Self-Reflection (Adapted for Nursing education)[12]
10.3 Develop capacity for leadership.		
10.3f Modify one's own leadership behaviors based on guided self-reflection.	AF4: Promote student self-evaluation skills	AF4: How do I know how my performance measures up when compared with assessment standards and competencies?
10.3 m Evaluate strategies/methods for peer review	AD1: Ensure robust procedures and processes in collaborative assessment	AD1: Do I have a good understanding of the assessment processes and requirements in nursing?
10.3n Participate in the evaluation of other members of the care team.	AD3: Ensure access and equal opportunity to participate in negotiated assessment options	AD3: Do I know how to access and use available resources and build networks to support my learning now and into the healthcare workplace?

Note. EAT dimensions are adapted for nursing education: AL = assessment literacy, AF = assessment feedback, AD = assessment design.

Assessment Literacy

Evans' Equity-Agency-Transparency (EAT) framework tool[9,10] integrates learning theory with practical application of assessment feedback in the classroom. The EAT framework is based on evidence from the literature on self-regulated learning and assessment literacy, feedback, and design. Tools and resources associated with the EAT framework emphasize assessments designed to foster student ownership of learning, metacognition, and management of emotions in a classroom culture of learning. Evans views students as "active contributors to the assessment feedback process rather than seeing assessment as something that is done to them."[9(p2)]

The EAT framework describes a classroom culture of learning based on three core concepts[10]:

- Equity—students experience feedback in a way that is understandable and accessible to all
- Agency—the student shares responsibility for assessment and learning with the instructor and peers
- Transparency—the assessment design and processes are clear to students ahead of time with no hidden components

The EAT framework is built on three core dimensions of practice, each having four practice areas, that can be viewed through the lens of nursing education and practice[11]:

- Assessment literacy (AL)—students and instructors understand and agree on what constitutes good performance and achievement of competencies
  - AL1: Clarify what constitutes "good" in nursing education and practice

- AL2: Explain how assessment elements are aligned or fit together
- AL3: Clarify the student role in assessment
- AL4: Define nursing- and specialty-specific competencies
- Assessment feedback—students act as feedback seekers who receive, use, and give feedback in a lifelong learning process
  - AF1: Provide accessible feedback students can understand and use for improvement
  - AF2: Provide early opportunities for students to receive and act on feedback
  - AF3: Prepare students to give and receive feedback to peers
  - AF4: Promote student self-evaluation skills
- Assessment design—instructors apply principles of universal design to create opportunities for triangulation of feedback from multiple sources
  - AD1: Ensure robust procedures and processes in collaborative assessment design
  - AD2: Promote meaningful, authentic assessment through real-world assessment opportunities
  - AD3: Ensure access and equal opportunity through negotiated and managed assessment options
  - AD4: Ensure ongoing evaluation through iterative assessment cycles

The EAT framework and the AACN essentials related to feedback have parallel concepts that support the inclusion of three types of feedback in formative assessments aimed at growth and development (see **Table 1**). Nurse educators can create a culture of learning rich with information about how to achieve competencies and continuously improve performance by focusing on the feedback component of assessment and its alignment of concepts from the AACN essentials and the EAT framework.

Three Sources of Feedback

By triangulating feedback from three key sources, students are empowered to make decisions about how their performance measures up to core competencies and standards, where they excel, and where they have room for improvement. High-quality feedback makes it possible for students to create an actionable plan for improvement. Three types of feedback support a culture of learning in the assessment process[3] and should be integrated into assessments whenever possible:

- Instructor feedback: instructor guidance and insight on assessments designed *for* learning, in addition to the assessment *of* learning
- Peer feedback: structured peer-to-peer dialogue on performance between students of similar levels of competence
- Self-reflective feedback: metacognition and self-reflection that supports a self-regulated approach to learning

Instructor Assessment

Instructor feedback plays a complementary role to peer feedback and self-reflection. Hsieh and Hill suggest that peer feedback is most useful in earlier stages of the assessment process (ie, formative assessments) and instructor feedback should be viewed as equal in value to peer feedback rather than playing a prioritized role in a hierarchical feedback structure.[13] The role of instructor feedback is to challenge arguments and bring clarity to student work after they have had a chance to test their ideas through peer evaluation and self-reflection. It is the instructor's responsibility to design assessments and build classroom cultures that support mutual respect and caring for others.[13,14] When feedback from instructors and peers is embedded in a classroom culture built on mutual trust and respect-worthy feedback givers, students are more likely to be receptive to feedback from others and work toward improving their performance.[14]

Rubrics are a helpful tool for setting expectations for students and making clear what standards must be met for mastery of an activity.[15] Rubrics can be used by instructors to provide actionable feedback and are often formatted with ratings in the column headers and criteria for performance in each row (**Fig. 1**). By using descriptors such as "Met," "Partially Met," and "Not Yet Met," the instructor can communicate to students via the rubric where benchmarks are met and where there is room for improvement. Though clear rubrics are time-consuming to create, they can expedite the grading process for instructors, especially when instructors use the institution's learning management system (LMS) rubric tool to provide feedback to students.

With advance planning, instructors can provide timely, supportive feedback as students complete asynchronous assessment tasks. For example, the instructor can write pre-determined feedback for each possible response option on a multiple-choice question on a quiz within the LMS. Quiz settings can be adjusted to allow students to view the questions they missed, and the feedback for each possible answer will display automatically (**Fig. 2**). In this way, instructors can provide context for each possible response option to help the student understand why the answer they chose was or was not the best response. To encourage continued engagement with the material, quizzes can also be set to allow multiple attempts so there is an incentive for students to read through the feedback and take the quiz again.

Students can also provide feedback to instructors via technology. Polling tools can gather real-time information on how well students are understanding the material.[16] Questions can be pre-built-in applications such as Poll Everywhere, TopHat , or Kahoot so that instructors can pause during a lesson to pose questions to students. Instructors can then view the students' responses immediately to gauge understanding and determine which topics might need further explanation. Making responses anonymous lowers the stakes for learners, which means they may be more willing to participate by responding. In this way, the instructor receives real-time information about student comprehension. If students are not understanding, the instructor can intervene immediately by providing additional explanation, while the concept is still

Blog rubric			
Criteria	**Ratings**		
Reading level	2 pts Met At or below an 8th grade reading level	1 pts Partially met At or below a 12th grade reading level	0 pts Not yet Reading level exceeds that of a high school education
Content	2 pts Met Information presented such that low literacy or low health literacy would not be an issue. Where appropriate, paragraph breaks and bulleted lists are used to increase understanding.	1 pts Partially met Appropriate language for a general audience, though more difficult to understand. At least 400 words.	0 pts Not yet Concepts are poorly explained, or uses excessive text or medical jargon. Fewer than 400 words or greater than 2,000 words.
Layout	2 pts Met Headings levels and font sizes used in a consistent manner to improve ease of reading. Colors are high contrast and represent a unifying theme.	1 pts Partially met Some but not all of the criteria for "met", that is at least one of the following is used to improve the layout: headings, fonts, or colors.	0 pts Not yet No attempt made to alter the layout
Image	2 pts Met Image(s) enhance the message of the text, and are appealing. Images reinforce positive aspects (or actions that can be taken) to address the issue, rather than using negative or scare tactics. Included images are labeled for reuse and attribution is included if required. Alt text is provided on each image.	1 pts Partially met Some but not all of the criteria for "met", that is at least one of the following: visually appealing image, image labeled for reuse, image includes alt text.	0 pts Not yet No image included, or an image the detracts from the message.

Fig. 1. "Rubric example in Canvas LMS."

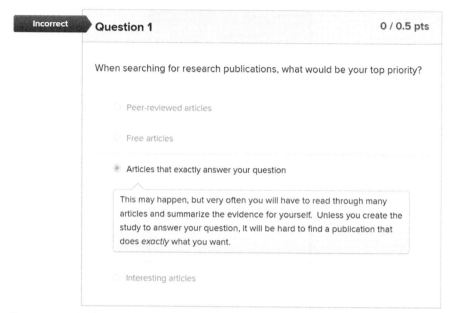

Fig. 2. "Example feedback on quiz question in Canvas LMS."

being explored, rather than later, after summative assessment reveals problems with comprehension.

Polling tools can also be used to improve student learning and retention by asking students to predict the answer to a question about instructional content before the content is taught.[17] Instead of polling students to check for understanding of a topic after it has been covered, instructors can ask students to anticipate the answer to a question or predict what happens next in a scenario. Evidence shows that even if students do not have prior knowledge about the topic, the act of predicting an answer and then learning the correct response helps students identify gaps in their knowledge.[18] By polling *before* teaching a concept, instructors are increasing the likelihood students will retain the information about to be presented. By polling *after* teaching a concept, instructors are giving students an opportunity for retrieval of information and practice.[17]

In addition to pre-determined questions, it is valuable to include opportunities for students to provide open-ended feedback to instructors. Survey tools such as Qualtrics, Google Forms , or Microsoft Forms can be used to create "exit tickets" for students to complete anonymously (**Fig. 3**). Using a URL shortener and QR code image, instructors include a link at the end of their presentation to an anonymous, open-ended survey that prompts students for any questions, comments, or concerns that they may have. By using a survey tool that automatically time-stamps each response, instructors can keep a running list of student queries and comments and respond to those questions during the next class session.

Peer Feedback

Feedback from instructors and peers, especially when it is combined with self-reflection, provides opportunities for performance improvement, practice with emotional regulation and communication skills, and development of professional maturity.[6] Increasing nurses' knowledge and use of supportive peer review processes enhances team performance and improves patient care outcomes.[19] Therefore,

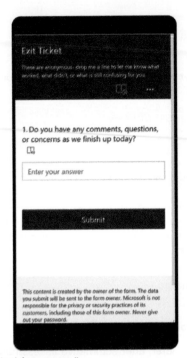

Fig. 3. "Example of an exit ticket survey."

including peer review instruction in nursing education courses and assessing the impact of peer review teaching strategies on student learning outcomes is essential. The feedback that results from a peer-review process in formative assessment provides a greater quantity of information from more diverse perspectives about where performance gaps exist and how improvement can be achieved. More importantly, when a student engages in evaluating a peer's work and providing feedback, they engage in a metacognitive, self-evaluative process that has benefits to their own learning.[20] A student who provides feedback begins to think more deeply about the standards against which they are reviewing their peer's work and how their own work measures up to those standards.[21]

Peer review works well in assessments of many kinds, including team performance, clinical or simulation performance, presentations, and written assignments. In all cases, students are better equipped to provide feedback to their peers when performance standards are clearly communicated. To assist students in providing high-quality supportive feedback to their peers, instructors should make explicit five characteristics of supportive feedback (**Box 1**) and explain to students how to integrate these into their feedback to peers. If students are confident that they can create supportive feedback for peers that is caring and aimed at growth, they are less likely to be afraid to be honest simply because their feedback is not anonymous.[22]

Instructors should provide students with a rubric for use during the peer review process that defines competencies and standards against which students compare their peer's work and provide feedback about what was done well and what can be improved. It is best practice to have students provide narrative feedback with no ratings or rankings to peers.[23] It is paramount that peer feedback not be used to assign grades or scores, as peer feedback works best as a formative approach to

---

Box 1
Five characteristics of supportive feedback

Supportive feedback for peers is

Focused. Feedback references standards or competencies related to practice and academic performance.

Descriptive. Feedback describes objective observations of what a peer reviewer can see, hear, or sense in the reviewee's performance.

Constructive. Feedback uses positive, sensitive language to inspire growth, even when feedback recommends improvement.

Blended. Feedback consists of a blend of specific observations of what is working well to meet standards and where the gaps are between the performance and the standards.

Achievable. Specific recommendations for closing performance gaps inspire the feedback receiver to move their performance to the next level. Achievable recommendations are not intended to move the feedback receiver from a low level of performance to the maximum level of performance in one feedback event. The expectation is that peer feedback helps the student move to the next higher level of competency, one benchmark at a time.

Note. Five characteristics of supportive feedback were developed by the first author and are based on a broad view of the literature.

---

assessment *for* learning, not a summative assessment *of* learning.[1] If instructors wish to assign points to the peer review activity, students should be graded on the quality of feedback they provide to peers rather than any quantitative interpretation of the feedback their peers provided.

Many LMSs include a peer review or peer feedback tool, and this feature can be used to facilitate the logistics of the peer feedback process. LMS feedback tools allow a rubric to be attached to the assignment within the LMS, and students can be reminded via the LMS to complete their reviews of their peers' work. If an LMS does not support peer review or provide robust functionality, other applications or learning technologies can be used. For written assignments, students can collaboratively author and comment on peers' work using cloud-based authoring tools such as Google Drive or Microsoft Office 365 using the "Comment" or "Suggest edit" features in Google Docs or Track Changes in Microsoft Word. Sharing of cloud-based documents can be one-to-one or one-to-many so that students work in pairs, small groups, or as an entire class group to provide feedback. Document sharing settings for cloud-based peer review should be set to protect privacy among student pairs or groups by requiring them to sign in before editing or providing peer feedback.

Self-Assessment and Reflection

A self-regulated approach to learning requires skills in self-assessment and the ability to reflect on and evaluate one's own performance. Students who can take a metacognitive approach to acquisition of competencies required for practice are able to independently identify achievement gaps and take action to close them.[3] Active learning strategies and frequent opportunities to practice skills in authentic contexts provide a rich environment in which students can monitor their own progress and continuously improve their practice[3]—an essential step in taking on a professional nursing identify.[7] Feedback from instructors and feedback from peers are equally important in nurturing students' development of self-evaluative judgment.[13] Students triangulate feedback information from peers, instructors, and their own metacognitive processes to engage in a comparison of their performance to educational or practice standards in a process of self-evaluative judgment.[14,21] In this way, they grow increasingly less dependent on instructor guidance to regulate their educational activities as they progress through their academic programs and begin to calibrate their own learning.

One approach to fostering self-assessment is to have students create the rubric for a given assignment.[24] Though students may be novices in creating rubrics, the instructor can guide class discussions around questions such as "What would the best example of [a task or assignment, for example, a public presentation] be? What do you think would be an example of an unacceptable effort?" With some prompting, students will provide the categories for what should (and should not) be present in the final product. The instructor can then organize the categories and descriptions created by the students into a rubric that they use to evaluate themselves. **Box 2** provides an example of a classroom activity to produce a rubric using this strategy.

Students can also review their performance on any hands-on task or patient interaction, such as demonstrations on simulated patients, by using video recordings. Over time, barriers to student creation of videos have diminished significantly because most student-owned smartphones have cameras and microphones adequate for this purpose. Professional audiovisual equipment is not required, and most students are sufficiently savvy with their personal devices to complete a recording, save it, and upload it to the institution's LMS.

DISCUSSION

Knowing when and how to use self-regulated learning strategies to achieve optimal individual and team effectiveness is key to the development of professionalism and leadership in nursing. Self-regulated learning depends on knowing how to seek feedback, process it cognitively and emotionally, and use it to achieve competency and improve performance. Courses designed to support the development of essential skills in self-regulation of learning equip students with skills in self-evaluative judgment. Nurse educators can use principles of competency-based education, AACN

Box 2
Example classroom process for student-created rubrics

The instructor can begin with a class discussion about public speaking and ask students to describe attributes of the best presentations they have seen, followed by characteristics of average presentations, and finally, what makes for the worst presentations. A grading rubric for an oral presentation is created from this dialogue with students. The instructor then tells the students they will be completing oral presentations in class to develop public speaking skills, and they will be grading themselves.

During the presentations, an iPad with camera and microphone (or webcam and microphone) can be used to record student presentations, and the instructor can then make the recordings available in the LMS for later review. Students can then review their recorded presentation and complete a self-evaluation on the rubric they created as a class. Given the anxiety many people have around public speaking, allowing students to evaluate themselves and discover where they have room for growth lowers the stakes for the activity.

For ease of compiling rubric responses, the grading rubric can be created in a survey tool such as Qualtrics, Google Forms, or Microsoft Forms. The form should prompt students for their first and last name, clearly display rubric criteria and ratings, and include open-ended questions or response fields to prompt deeper self-reflection. An example of a rubric for this assignment is in **Fig. 4.**

The first category is **"what you say"**. As a class we determined the following definitions:

Bad presentation	Best presentation
Jumping around topics "Um" or "like" Speaking too fast	Logical sequence of information Appropriate tone and emphasis Good pacing

How well did you do with **what you said?**

Needs improvement   Acceptable   Best presentation

The second category is **body language**. As a class we determined the following definitions:

Bad presentation	Best presentation
Blinking like crazy or looking down Fidgeting or swaying Movement that detracts from the message	Maintain eye contact Meaningful hand gestures Engaged with audience

How well did you do with **body language**?

Needs improvement   Acceptable   Best presentation

The third category is **preparation**. As a class we determined the following definitions:

Bad presentation	Best presentation
Not enough information Obvious lack of knowledge on topic Sounds scripted or is reading from a script	Enough information is provided Conversational while also getting to the point Knows the audience

How well did you do with **preparation**?

Needs improvement   Acceptable   Best presentation

The fourth category is **confidence**. As a class we determined the following definitions:

Bad presentation	Best presentation
Voice cracks Visibly nervous Repetition	Authoritative Confident Personable

How well did you do with **confidence**?

Needs improvement   Acceptable   Best presentation

For the remaining points, reflect on what you learned as part of this process. What went well? What didn't go well? What will you remember to do the next time you present?

Any other comments or feedback about this activity?

Fig. 4. "Rubric for self-evaluation of oral presentation".

Essentials focused on feedback, and the EAT framework to design formative assessment process with multiple sources of internal and external feedback.

Student capacity to assume leadership roles in building healthy communities, reducing health disparities, and caring for patients and families will depend in part on their ability to skillfully communicate supportive feedback to peers and colleagues.[25] Thus, it is critical that students are presented with opportunities in the academic setting to practice soliciting and acting on peer feedback regarding their own personal strengths and weaknesses in addition to providing supportive feedback to peers.

Learning technologies that are especially helpful in providing opportunities to take up feedback from external sources and internal reflective processes include peer-review and rubric tools in LMSs, survey tools, videography using institutional equipment or students' personal devices, and audience response systems. Challenges include a potential learning process for both faculty and students to become comfortable with educational technology, cost of learning applications or digital equipment and resources, and time required to design learning activities, create rubrics, and upload content to digital applications. These challenges can be mitigated by intentionally choosing learning technologies supported by the educational institution and identifying reliable instructional technology support available to faculty and students. The effort required to design or redesign formative assessments that generate multiple sources of feedback will be recovered in rich, engaging assessment experiences focused on learning and meaningful feedback that drives competency achievement and performance improvement.

SUMMARY

Achievement of essential nursing competencies is facilitated by a culture of learning in which assessment is designed as a developmental process co-created by faculty and students, with an open dialogue and an emphasis on coaching rather than judgment. In the assessment for learning, three key sources of feedback—instructor, peer, and self—are triangulated to provide critical information the student needs for continuous improvement and, ultimately, performance of core competencies at a level appropriate for summative assessment. Developing a deeper understanding of peer-to-peer feedback processes will prepare students to develop metacognitive approaches to learning and facilitate the achievement of core competencies while practicing peer-to-peer feedback skills necessary for nursing practice. Nurse educators can support assessment for learning and help students triangulate multiple sources of feedback for growth by incorporating peer review assignments in academic experiences and using learning technologies to facilitate the learning process.

CLINICS CARE POINTS

- A classroom culture of learning depends on formative assessments that provide feedback from the instructor and peers in combination with opportunities for self-reflection.
- Grading rubrics, polling strategies, and automated quiz feedback promote rich and timely instructor feedback through technology.
- Supportive peer review processes are key to providing feedback to students from multiple perspectives and in greater quantities than an instructor alone can provide.
- Self-assessment and reflection allow students to triangulate feedback information and make decisions about how to achieve competencies and close gaps in performance.

- Technology-supported teaching strategies such as peer review, polling, videography, and surveys promote formative approaches to assessment that facilitate learning.

DISCLOSURE

The authors have nothing to disclose.

REFERENCES

1. Brand PLP, Jaarsma ADC, van der Vleuten CPM. Driving lesson or driving test? A metaphor to help faculty separate feedback from assessment. Perspect Med Educ 2021;10(1):50–6.
2. Broadbent J, Panadero E, Boud D. Implementing summative assessment with a formative flavour: a case study in a large class. Assess Eval Higher Education 2018;43(2):307–22.
3. Evans C, Waring M. Enhancing students' assessment feedback skills within higher education. Oxford Research Encyclopedia of Education; 2020. Available at: https://oxfordre.com/education/view/10.1093/acrefore/9780190264093.001. 0001/acrefore-9780190264093-e-932. Accessed March 3, 2022.
4. Panadero E, Broadbent J, Boud D. Using formative assessment to influence self- and co-regulated learning: the role of evaluative judgement. Eur J Psychol Educ 2019;34:535–57.
5. Ata AA, Abdelwahid AE. Nursing students' metacognitive thinking and goal orientation as predictors of academic motivation. Am J Nurs Res 2019;7(5):793–801.
6. Altmiller G, Deal B, Ebersole N, et al. Constructive feedback teaching strategy: a multisite study of its effectiveness. Nurs Educ Perspect 2018;39(5):291–6.
7. American Association of Colleges of Nursing (AACN). The essentials: core competencies for professional nursing education. AACN. 2021. Available at: https:// www.aacnnursing.org/Portals/42/AcademicNursing/pdf/Essentials-2021.pdf. Accessed March 4, 2022.
8. American Association of Colleges of Nursing (AACN). Competency-based education and assessment. Document download from the Professional and advanced nursing education essentials tool kit. 2021. Available at: https://www. aacnnursing.org/Portals/42/Downloads/Essentials/CBE-Draft.pdf; https://www. aacnnursing.org/AACN-Essentials/Implementation-Tool-Kit. Accessed March 9, 2022.
9. Evans C. Enhancing assessment feedback practice in higher education: the EAT framework. 2016. Available at: https://www.southampton.ac.uk/assets/imported/ transforms/content-block/UsefulDownloads_Download/ A0999D3AF2AF4C5AA24B5BEA08C61D8E/EAT%20Guide%20April%20FINAL 1%20ALL.pdf.
10. Evans C. EAT Framework. Available at: https://www.eatframework.com/. Accessed March 4, 2022.
11. Evans C. EAT Framework – Instructor. Available at: https://www.eatframework. com/instructors. Accessed March 4, 2022.
12. Evans C. EAT Framework – Student. Available at: https://www.eatframework.com/ students-1. Accessed March 4, 2022.
13. Hsieh YC, Hill C. Reconceptualizing the value of peer and instructor feedback using a sequential structure. Assess Eval Higher Education 2021;26:1–4.

14. Fong CJ, Schallert DL, Williams KM, et al. When feedback signals failure but offers hope for improvement: a process model of constructive criticism. Thinking Skills and Creativity 2018;30:42–53.

15. Balloo K, Evans C, Hughes A, et al. Transparency isn't spoon-feeding: how a transformative approach to the use of explicit assessment criteria can support student self-regulation. Front Education 2018;3:69.

16. Herrada RI, Baños R, Alcayde A. Student response systems: a multidisciplinary analysis using visual analytics. Education Sci 2020;10(12):348.

17. Brod G. Predicting as a learning strategy. Psychon Bull Rev 2021;28(6):1839–47.

18. Lang JM. Small teaching: everyday lessons from the Science of learning. 2nd edition. Jossey-Bass; 2021.

19. Herrington CR, Hand MW. Impact of nurse peer review on a culture of safety. J Nurs Care Qual 2019;34(2):158–62.

20. Nicol D, Thomson A, Breslin C. Rethinking feedback practices in higher education: a peer review perspective. Assess Eval Higher Education 2014;39(1): 102–22.

21. Yan Z, Carless D. Self-assessment is about more than self: the enabling role of feedback literacy. Assess Eval Higher Education 2021;1:1–3.

22. Haag-Heitman B, George V. Peer review in nursing: principles for successful practice. Sudbury, MA: Jones and Bartlett; 2011.

23. Wanner T, Palmer E. Formative self- and peer assessment for improved student learning: the crucial factors of design, teacher participation and feedback. Assess Eval Higher Education 2018;43(7):1032–47.

24. Evans C. EAT Framework Appendix F: Student Role in Assessment. 2020. Available at: https://app.secure.griffith.edu.au/exlnt/entry/9669/view. Accessed March 9, 2020.

25. Morse V, Warshawsky NE. Nurse leader competencies: today and tomorrow. Nurs Adm Q 2021;45(1):65–70.

Teaching Strategies for Online Nurse Practitioner Physical Assessment and Telehealth Education

Heidi Bobek, DNP, APRN-CNP*

KEYWORDS

- Curricula • Distance education • Nurse practitioner • Nursing education
- Physical examination • Program evaluation • Telemedicine • Videoconferencing

KEY POINTS

- Physical assessment skills can be taught in an online environment and result in student achievement of learning outcomes equal to those achieved with in-person instruction.
- Multimodal teaching strategies (lecture, laboratory and simulation, clinical experiences, and projects) are essential for online learning of physical assessment skills and telehealth competencies.
- Professional nursing organizations and national health care organizations support the incorporation of telehealth into nurse practitioner education.
- Helpful telehealth resources are available online for health care providers and nursing faculty to support telehealth education and practice.

INTRODUCTION

During the coronavirus disease (COVID-19) pandemic, in response to a need to rapidly transition nursing education to the online environment, faculty turned to technology and online teaching strategies supported by nursing education research to keep students engaged. Nursing faculty in advanced physical assessment courses were especially challenged in the transition to online coursework, and sustained student engagement through evidence-based strategies for teaching physical assessment skills, such as video for teaching and evaluation, student self-reflection, and provision of feedback from multiple sources.[1] Virtual simulation in physical assessment instruction also presented an alternative to replace in-person physical assessment laboratories based on evidence of the effectiveness of virtual simulation in the achievement of learning outcomes and student satisfaction.[2]

The Ohio State University College of Nursing, Columbus, 1585 Neil Avenue, Columbus, OH 43210, USA
* Corresponding author.
E-mail address: bobek.7@osu.edu

Nurs Clin N Am 57 (2022) 589–598
https://doi.org/10.1016/j.cnur.2022.07.003
0029-6465/22/© 2022 Elsevier Inc. All rights reserved.

Moreover, during the pandemic, graduate nursing students suddenly found themselves learning to navigate the telehealth environment and conduct a physical assessment virtually. In some cases, their clinical preceptors were learning to use telehealth applications and conduct patient-assisted telehealth assessments alongside the students. For example, to assess respiratory status, instead of auscultating the lungs with a stethoscope, a health care provider must work within the virtual environment of the telehealth application to observe the patient skin color, watch for the rise and fall of the chest, listen for audible wheezing, and watch for the patient to become short of breath while speaking in complete sentences. This transition to virtual approaches to physical assessment was new for some practitioners as well as students.

There is evidence that telehealth has had a positive impact on increased access to quality care and increased patient satisfaction, and health care organizations are likely to continue to expand post-pandemic telehealth services for all patient populations.[3] Inclusion of technology and telehealth is identified as a key competency for nurse practitioners and an important content area by the National Organization of Nurse Practitioner Faculties (NONPF).[4] Further expansion of high-quality telehealth education in health care curricula is essential to developing advanced practice providers who are ready to practice in a dynamic and challenging health care delivery environment.[5] This calls for adaptations of advanced physical assessment education that ensure flexible online instruction and incorporation of telehealth skills and competencies to provide effective telehealth care.

ONLINE PHYSICAL ASSESSMENT EDUCATION

Health care providers are taught early in their training that the utilization of effective communication skills and the art of gathering a detailed patient history are powerful tools when assessing a patient. Obtaining a thorough patient history, including history of present illness, past medical history, social history, family history, medications, allergies, and surgeries/hospitalizations often leads the health care provider to a particular diagnosis or several sound differential diagnoses. A diagnosis is often subsequently confirmed after performing a focused physical examination. Online physical assessment education can be just as effective in teaching skills and competencies required for physical assessment as in-person education when using evidence-based teaching strategies.

It is important to note that while there are many studies suggesting increased confidence and effective learning outcomes for students participating in online physical assessment courses, there is little empirical support for specific, evidence-based approaches to teaching physical assessment skills online, especially with the integration of telehealth techniques. While online education is not a new concept, there are new challenges in determining best practices because of the rapid, pandemic-related transition to online education and the dynamic nature of learning and practice technologies. What follows is a review of the literature on teaching strategies in online physical assessment education for advanced practice nurses that informs current and future approaches to teaching strategies, technology, and modes of instruction.

Peer Review of Video Skill Demonstrations

A retrospective study compared a traditional, in-person physical assessment course to an online physical assessment course and measured outcomes related to skills readiness in advanced practice nursing students.[1] Both courses incorporated curricular elements of didactic content, skills practice, history taking, skill demonstration feedback, and final evaluation of skills. The traditional course used textbook readings, video reviews, in-person lectures, and student demonstration of skills to student peers with immediate feedback from faculty and laboratory partners. Skills were practiced at home as well as in-person on campus, and a final evaluation of skills was performed on a standardized patient. Feedback on skills included in-person faculty critique during laboratory practice and feedback from the student laboratory partner.

In contrast, the online course used textbook readings and video demonstrations from the publisher but also included a video created by a previous student demonstrating physical assessment skills outside of a laboratory setting. Students practiced skills at home, and they practiced history taking and clinical reasoning skills in videoconferencing tools. They recorded their physical assessment on a volunteer, self-assessed their video, and received feedback on the video from two-course peers and faculty.

The online approach showed that there was no statistically significant difference between their final physical examination assessment in the traditional in-person course and the online course. Students reported satisfaction with faculty feedback and cited peer review of videos as the most helpful element of their learning in the online course.[1]

Low-Fidelity Online Physical Assessment Laboratories

Another study focused on a fully online physical assessment course that included an online asynchronous physical assessment laboratory with low-fidelity simulation and peer feedback.[6] Students recorded themselves practicing system-specific focused physical assessments on a significant other or manikin. Students then reviewed their peers' recorded videos and provided feedback using a skills checklist. The faculty also provided narrative feedback on each video. Students were also required to complete a full head-to-toe comprehensive physical assessment at the end of the class to pass the course. Evaluation of the course utilized the Kirkpatrick model of evaluation.[7] This model, often used with simulation, suggests learning from training programs at four levels:

- Reaction—Do learners find the training engaging and relevant to their future work?
- Learning—Are required knowledge, skills, and attitudes (competencies) being met?
- Behavior—Are students applying what they learned through behavioral change?
- Results—Are patient and organizational outcomes being met?[7]

The study revealed that 78% of students felt the course was as effective as the in-person physical assessment course taken previously in the prelicensure nursing program; 89% of students reported that the course prepared them for the comprehensive head-to-toe assessment, and 78% of students agreed that the self-recorded practice with peer feedback as well as providing peer feedback to others improved their physical assessment skills.[6]

Local Tutors and Proprietary Virtual Simulation Applications

Another study explored the combination of virtual web-based simulation and program feedback, incorporation of a local tutor, and optional in-person skills laboratory for online delivery of a physical assessment course.[8] Students were required to participate in weekly cases in Shadow Health, an online virtual simulation program, to perform a focused physical examination on a standardized digital patient, after which they received software-generated feedback in Shadow Health. Assessment results in Shadow Health were also available to faculty who could provide additional feedback if needed. Students were required to meet with a local tutor or advanced practice provider (nurse practitioner (NP), clinical nurse specialist (CNS), physician assistant (PA), doctor of medicine (MD), doctor of osteopathic medicine (DO)) on a regular basis for a professional evaluation of the students' physical assessment skills and verbal feedback. Additionally, students were offered two separate in-person skills laboratories to practice and receive faculty feedback; however, only a small number of students attended the optional laboratories (10% of students attended the first laboratory while 14% of students attended the second skills laboratory). All students passed a 30-minute comprehensive physical examination performed on an adult person under faculty or local tutor observation with a 90% competency rate.[8]

Social Learning in Virtual Patient Environments

A quasi-experimental study of 40 senior nursing students provided evidence to support the use of a social learning approach, the ability to learn through observation with future use of the modeled behavior, along with the implementation of a cloud-based virtual patient program enhanced student learning, self-efficacy, and communication skills with automated program feedback and guidance. Students also felt the virtual patient environment made learning more enjoyable.[9]

It is important to note that these studies incorporated various forms of multisource feedback. Multisource feedback includes self-assessment, faculty feedback, and peer feedback to enhance the student experience and build metacognitive skills through formative assessment and learning.[10]

TELEHEALTH EDUCATION AND RESOURCES

After students achieve competency in basic physical assessment skills, the next challenge involves the act of performing a physical assessment within telehealth visits. Telehealth is defined by the Health Resources and Services Administration as "the use of electronic information and telecommunication technologies to support long-distance clinical health care, patient and professional health-related education, health administration, and public health." These technologies include the Internet, video conferencing, streaming media, and land and wireless communications.[11]

Advantages of telehealth include improved access to care, improved patient satisfaction, and positive health outcomes.[3] A prepandemic 2015 Cochrane review[12] looked at 93 randomized controlled trials with over 22,000 participants that focused on interactive telemedicine effects on health care outcomes. The results found no differences in heart failure patients treated in person versus patients treated via telemedicine. Moreover, telemedicine treatment resulted in improved glucose control in some diabetic patients, decreased blood pressure in some patients, and no significant difference in outcomes for patients with mental health or substance abuse problems.[12] The no-show rate for patient visits also dramatically decreased as telehealth utilization increased.[13] According to the US Department of Health and Human Services, Medicare utilization of telehealth increased 63-fold during the pandemic,[14] and predictions suggest that telehealth visits will continue to account for approximately 20% of all health care visits post-pandemic.[15]

When in-person physical examinations are not possible, virtual patient visits via telehealth technology provide an alternative means to deliver care, but they also present a challenge to providers who lack telehealth skills. In response to the significant increase in telehealth delivery during the COVID-19 pandemic, telehealth experts and professional organizations identified, described, and disseminated resources to support virtual physical assessment for health care providers to use and adapt to serve their patient population via telehealth. For example, a primary care telehealth visit focusing on hypertension will be different than an orthopedic specialty telehealth visit focusing on an ankle injury. Recommendations related to the orthopedic telehealth examination include providing verbal instructions to the patient in layman's terms, such as "lift your lower leg into the view of the camera and move your ankle in a circle" before and during the virtual visit and having patients watch a video on a split screen during the visit.[16] The health care provider can assess the skin color, signs of swelling or bruising, and assess joint range of motion when providing the patient with these instructions. In contrast, a telehealth assessment for hypertension might include instructing the patient to "move your neck into the view of the camera" for the health care provider to assess for jugular vein distention. Instructing the patient to "move legs into the view of the camera and then use your thumb to press into the skin of the lower leg" allows the health care provider to assess lower extremity skin color, signs of swelling, and pitting edema. Health care providers can also ask to view a patient's written blood pressure log or observe the patient taking their blood pressure using an at-home monitor. For pediatric telehealth visits, Children's Health of Orange County developed a tip sheet specifically for the physical assessment of pediatric patients.[17] Another example of a resource for telehealth providers who conduct physical assessments is the Telehealth Ten,[18] a set of 10 steps for a patient-assisted virtual physical examination (**Fig. 1**). This 10-step checklist is intended for use during the physical examination of patients with chronic diseases and emphasizes the cardiovascular system. The Telehealth Ten checklist can easily be adapted to other body systems or specialties during a telehealth visit. Additional virtual physical assessment resources to assist advanced practice providers and nurse educators with telehealth education and practice are listed in **Table 1**.

TELEHEALTH EDUCATION CURRICULA

In 2018, NONPF recommended the inclusion of telehealth technology in the nurse practitioner curriculum to support the NONPF Technology and Information Literacy Competency.[4] Recommendations for teaching strategies and curricula include didactic content, simulation, and standardized patients, and clinical experiences.[19] Suggested telehealth competencies to guide curricular development include:

- Telehealth etiquette and professionalism while videoconferencing
- Skills in using peripherals, such as an otoscope, stethoscope, and ophthalmoscope
- An understanding of when telehealth should or should not be used
- An understanding of privacy and protected health information regulations
- Proficiency in the use of synchronous and asynchronous telehealth technology
- Knowledge of appropriate documentation and billing of telehealth technology
- An ability to collaborate interprofessionally using telehealth technologies
- Proficiency in taking a history, performing an appropriate physical examination, and generating differential diagnoses using telehealth[19]

A 2021 systematic review focused on the integration of telehealth training into health care provider education found many differences between the curricula in different programs.[5] For instance, one program required telehealth training while it was optional for others. One telehealth training session lasted for 1 hour while another training consisted of a weekend immersion followed by an 8-hour clinical experience. Overall, all of the nurse-practitioner programs reported high student satisfaction with the telehealth training, but the authors found no empirical studies based on objective data in

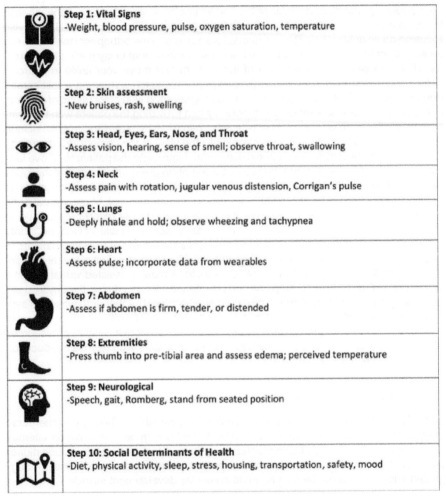

Fig. 1. The Telehealth ten checklist is an example of a tool than can assist health care providers to perform physical examinations during telehealth visits.

the review that included evidence-based guidelines for integration of telehealth education in physical assessment curricula.[5]

A guide for telehealth education focuses on the four Ps of the Telehealth framework (planning, preparing, providing, and performance evaluation)[19] which provides a model for integrating telehealth competencies. This guide recommends a multimodal approach to practitioner telehealth education based upon the four Ps framework that includes didactic education, simulation, clinical education, and student projects **(Fig. 2)**.

DISCUSSION

Various educational strategies are available to teach physical assessment of a patient in an online health care education program. Evidence-based instructional strategies include lecture-based content, student self-recorded videos of skills to demonstrate

Table 1
Resources for telehealth providers and educators

Resources	Descriptions
Center for Telehealth, Innovation, Education, and Research (C-TIER) (https://telehealtheducation-ctier.com/news-and-resources)	• Videos demonstrating simulated telehealth visits obtaining a health history, focused physical assessment, and discussion of findings • Two-week self-paced telehealth certification course • Recommendations for incorporating telehealth in nursing education • Current policy, white papers, and innovation focused on telehealth
NONPF Telehealth Portal (https://www.nonpf.org/page/TeleResources)	• NONPF membership required for access • Telehealth toolkits, nursing faculty development, telehealth platforms, billing/regulation/policy information, interprofessional collaboration, ethics/health equity • Recommendations for incorporating telehealth in nursing education
National Consortium of Telehealth Resource Centers (https://telehealthresourcecenter.org/)	• Telehealth basics, fact sheets, state laws governing telehealth practices, education webinars, toolkits • Federally Qualified Health Care resources focused on rural and underserved communities • Meets NONPF telehealth competencies
Centers for Medicare and Medicaid (https://www.cms.gov/files/document/telehealth-toolkit- providers.pdf)	• Telehealth basics • Tips for getting started with telehealth • Working with special populations (eg, people with disabilities, non-English speaking patients, rural populations, behavioral health) • Federal (Medicare) and State (Medicaid) billing policies • Documentation and coding tips • Technical assistance/resources
The Bates' Visual Guide of Physical Assessment (https://batesvisualguide-com)	• Physical assessment skill videos for each body system • Physical assessment skill videos for pediatric body systems • Head-to-toe assessment videos • Over 8 h of content
Caravan Health's Telehealth Physical Exam Guide (https://www.caltrc.org/get-started/telehealth-physical-exam-fact-sheet-caravan-health/)	• Cheat sheet for telehealth physical assessment for health care providers • Separate body systems
Children's Hospital of Orange County (https://www.choc.org/telehealth-resources/)	• Virtual physical examination guide • Specific to pediatrics

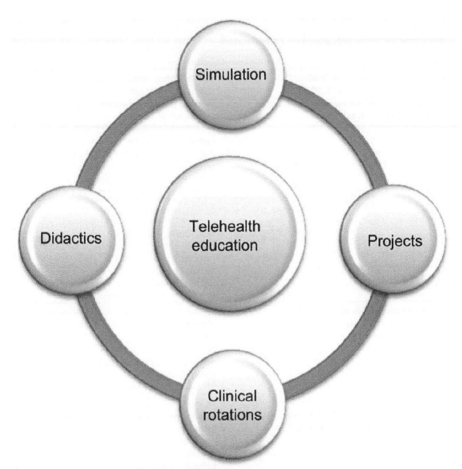

Fig. 2. The four Ps framework is an effective model to guide health care provider telehealth education. Reproduced with permission by Dr. Carolyn Rutledge PhD, FNP-BC. First published at Rutledge, C. M., Kott, K., Schweickert, P., Poston, R., Fowler, C., Haney, T. (2017). "Telehealth and eHealth in Nurse Practitioner Training: Current Perspectives". Advances in Medical Educations and Practice. 8, 399-409.

competency of physical assessment, and peer and faculty feedback on student skills videos. While the literature describes positive learning outcomes and increased student confidence with physical assessment skills when using these strategies, more research is needed to determine best practices in online training in physical assessment, especially with reference to effective approaches to teaching physical assessment techniques in a telehealth environment.

Relaxed billing practices and HIPAA regulations during the pandemic allowed for a significant increase in telehealth visits, and unexpected benefits and challenges of telehealth emerged as a result. The American Academy of Family Physicians published an opinion article encouraging four main changes to telehealth that should be sustained post-pandemic: (1) increased HIPAA flexibility, for example, allowing Facetime and Zoom to complete a virtual visit; (2) continuation of Medicare and Medicaid policies allowing telehealth for new patient visits and visits for all (not just for those in rural areas) and audio-only visits; (3) licensure in multiple states for physicians to increase telehealth access; and (4) prescription of controlled substances following a telehealth visit.[20] Advocacy and research exploring outcomes of current practices will likely be required for these changes to become permanent in health care delivery in the future.

SUMMARY

Regardless of how policies ultimately regulate virtual health care delivery, telehealth services delivered by nurse practitioners are likely to expand in the future. Nurses need to prepare to respond by developing, evaluating, researching, and refining curricula in virtual patient care. Specifically, nurse practitioner students need opportunities to incorporate their new physical assessment skills into a virtual telehealth environment to conduct a successful virtual patient visit. Utilization of the four Ps of the Telehealth framework provides comprehensive integration of telehealth competencies in advanced nurse practitioner education.

CLINICS CARE POINTS

- Nursing students find online physical assessment courses a positive and meaningful experience in their nursing education.
- Evidence-based recommendations and guides are available for performing and documenting a physical assessment during a telehealth visit.
- Utilization of the four Ps of telehealth is an effective strategy for the incorporation of telehealth into nurse practitioner education.
- Telehealth resources are available online for health care providers and nursing faculty to use in educational and clinical settings.
- Gaps in knowledge related to telehealth and physical assessment education present robust opportunities for nurses to engage in scholarship.

DISCLOSURE

The author has nothing to disclose.

REFERENCES

1. Higgins K, Kirkland T, Le-Jenkins U, et al. Preparing students to be ready for practice: An innovative approach to teaching advanced physical assessment skills online. J Am Assoc Nurse Pract 2019;31(11):640–7.
2. Padilha JM, Machado PP, Ribeiro A, et al. Clinical Virtual Simulation in Nursing Education: Randomized Controlled Trial. J Med Internet Res 2019;21(3):e11529.
3. Ramaswamy A, Yu M, Drangsholt S, et al. Patient Satisfaction With Telemedicine During the COVID-19 Pandemic: Retrospective Cohort Study. J Med Internet Res 2020;22(9):e20786.
4. NONPF Statement in Support of Telehealth in NP Education - National Organization of Nurse Practitioner Faculties (NONPF). Available at: https://www.nonpf.org/news/news.asp?id=388719&hhSearchTerms=%22telehealth%22. Accessed January 10, 2022.
5. Chike-Harris KE, Durham C, Logan A, et al. Integration of Telehealth Education into the Health Care Provider Curriculum: A Review. Telemed E-health 2021;27(2):137–49.

6. Webber-Ritchey KJ, Badowski D, Gibbons L. An Online Asynchronous Physical Assessment Lab (OAPAL) for Graduate Nursing Students Using Low-Fidelity Simulation With Peer Feedback. Nurs Educ Perspect 2020;41(6):378–9.

7. Johnston S, Coyer FM, Nash R. Kirkpatrick's Evaluation of Simulation and Debriefing in Health Care Education: A Systematic Review. J Nurs Educ 2018;57(7): 393–8.

8. Pickett S. Options for Teaching Physical Assessment Skills On-Line for Nurse Education Students. Teach Learn Nurs 2017;12(1):32–4.

9. Hwang GJ, Chang CY, Ogata H. The effectiveness of the virtual patient-based social learning approach in undergraduate nursing education: A quasi-experimental study. Nurse Educ Today 2022;108:105164.

10. Bonnel W, Boehm H. Improving Feedback to Students Online: Teaching Tips From Experienced Faculty. J Contin Educ Nurs 2011;42(11):503–9.

11. What is Telehealth? Official web site of the U.S. Health Resources & Services Administration. 2021. Available at: https://www.hrsa.gov/rural-health/telehealth/what-is-telehealth. Accessed December 31, 2021.

12. Flodgren G, Rachas A, Farmer AJ, et al. Interactive telemedicine: effects on professional practice and health care outcomes. Cochrane Database Syst Rev 2015; 9. https://doi.org/10.1002/14651858.CD002098.pub2.

13. Diegel-Vacek L, Cotler K, Reising V, et al. Transition of Nurse Practitioner Faculty Practice and Student Clinicals to Telehealth: Response to the COVID-19 Pandemic. J Nurse Pract 2021;17(3):317–21.

14. Division N. New HHS Study Shows 63-Fold Increase in Medicare Telehealth Utilization During the Pandemic. HHS.gov. 2021. Available at: https://www.hhs.gov/about/news/2021/12/03/new-hhs-study-shows-63-fold-increase-in-medicare-telehealth-utilization-during-pandemic.html. Accessed December 29, 2021.

15. Telemedicine Improves Care Across Johns Hopkins Medicine. Available at: https://www.hopkinsmedicine.org/news/articles/telemedicine-improves-care-across-johns-hopkins-medicine. Accessed December 29, 2021.

16. Lamplot JD, Pinnamaneni S, Swensen-Buza S, et al. The Virtual Shoulder and Knee Physical Examination. Orthop J Sports Med 2020;8(10). 2325967120962869.

17. CHOC. Children's Health Orange County. Available at: https://www.choc.org/. Accessed January 12, 2022.

18. Benziger CP, Huffman MD, Sweis RN, et al. The Telehealth Ten: A Guide for a Patient-Assisted Virtual Physical Examination. Am J Med 2021;134(1):48–51.

19. Rutledge CM, Kott K, Schweickert PA, et al. Telehealth and eHealth in nurse practitioner training: current perspectives. Adv Med Educ Pract 2017;8:399–409.

20. North S. These Four Telehealth Changes Should Stay, Even After the Pandemic. Fam Pract Manag 2021;28(3):9–11.

Disaster Preparedness

Keeping Nursing Staff and Students at the Ready

Todd E. Tussing, DNP, RN, CENP, NEA-BC[a,b,*],
Holly Chesnick, MS, RN, NE-BC[c,d], Amy Jackson, MS, RN, CNL, NE-BC[e,f]

KEYWORDS

- Continuing education • Crowdsourcing • Nursing students • Disaster planning
- Mass casualty incidents • Natural disasters • Simulation training • Virtual reality

KEY POINTS

- Declared disasters are increasing worldwide.
- A disaster preparedness conceptual model can serve as a guide for the development of disaster preparedness plans and disaster preparedness curriculum.
- Staff nurses should be in a state of continual disaster preparation.
- Staff and student nurse disaster preparation training should include the disaster plan, first aid, and disaster management.
- Technology supports successful disaster preparation training and disaster management.

BACKGROUND

Disasters leading to loss of life and property have been occurring in human societies since the beginning of recorded history. Disasters take a toll on those inflicted, striking all social, economic, and racial groups with little to no warning, and can last hours to months at a time. Health care organizations, specifically hospitals, can also be a victim of disaster events, including natural disasters (eg, weather events), man-made disasters (eg, mass shootings, cyberattacks), and disasters of circumstances (eg, power

[a] College of Nursing, The Ohio State University, 1585 Neil Avenue, Columbus, OH 43210, USA; [b] East Hospital, Wexner Medical Center at The Ohio State University, 181 Taylor Avenue, Columbus, OH 43202, USA; [c] Ambulatory Services, Wexner Medical Center at The Ohio State University, Suite 130, 650Ackerman Road, Columbus, OH 43202, USA; [d] Tower 5 Cardiology Inpatient Unit, East Hospital, Wexner Medical Center at The Ohio State University, 181 Taylor Avenue, Columbus, OH 43202, USA; [e] Ambulatory Services, Wexner Medical Center at The Ohio State University, Suite 3100, 2050 Kenney Road, Columbus, OH 43221, USA; [f] Tower 7 Medical-Surgical Inpatient Unit, East Hospital, Wexner Medical Center at The Ohio State University, 181 Taylor Avenue, Columbus, OH 43202, USA
* Corresponding author. College of Nursing, The Ohio State University, 1585 Neil Avenue, Columbus, OH 43210.
E-mail address: Tussing.9@osu.edu

Nurs Clin N Am 57 (2022) 599–611
https://doi.org/10.1016/j.cnur.2022.06.008
0029-6465/22/© 2022 Elsevier Inc. All rights reserved.

failures or internal floods). The generally unpredictable nature of disaster continues to impact our health care systems and populations worldwide.

Health care organizations have an ethical responsibility to act when disasters occur to provide immediate care to the sick or injured and, in the longer term, help stabilize the community in which they reside. Disaster preparedness is essential to hospital readiness to respond in a crisis. National regulations require hospitals to assess for disaster vulnerability and prepare a disaster plan for use during a crisis.[1] All hospital staff members, including providers, must be ready with the knowledge of the hospital disaster plan and their role within it.

Regulations and Standards

After the events of September 11, 2001, when a group of terrorists attacked the World Trade Center, the United States increased its efforts in the development of disaster preparation.[2] Health care organizations participating in Medicare billing, including hospitals, are required to meet the standards put forth by the Center for Medicare and Medicaid Services (CMS). Those standards are assessed by an external regulatory body for hospital compliance and reported back to CMS as a condition of participation in Medicare billing. In 2016, the CMS issued the *Emergency Preparedness Requirements for Medicare and Medicaid Participating Providers and Suppliers Final Rule* to establish emergency preparedness by health care organizations for disasters.[1] Following the announcement of CMS standards, The Joint Commission, a regulatory body with a mission to survey hospitals for CMS Regulatory compliance, began to survey hospitals for compliance with that rule after November of 2017. In addition to its survey function, The Joint Commission provides resources to health care providers to aid in the assessment of vulnerability and development of a disaster plan.[3]

Recognizing the critical role nurses play in disaster management, leaders in academia incorporated disaster preparation into educational standards for the nursing curriculum. The American Association for College of Nursing (AACN) released new core competencies in 2021 for undergraduate and graduate-level education that incorporated disaster preparation under Domain 3, Population Health.[4] Competencies for undergraduate and graduate nursing students involving disaster preparation are listed under Essential 3.6, Advance Preparedness to Protect Population Health During Disasters and Public Health Emergencies.[4] Literature showing the need for disaster preparation for nurses has also been published in Europe, Asia, Middle East, and the Pacific Islands and covers topics of preparation for both practicing nurses and nursing students.[5–7] Furthermore, the International Council of Nurses (ICN) published *Core Competencies in Disaster Nursing,* establishing consensus on the definition of disaster nursing, the role of the nurse in disasters, and competencies to guide nursing leaders and educators in disaster preparation for nurses.[8]

Role of the Hospital in Disaster Management

Disaster management has four phases: preparedness, mitigation, response, and recovery.[9] Hospitals, as a member of their community, play a role in each of the phases. The preparedness phase involves both an external and internal organizational assessment of the vulnerability of disasters, the development of a disaster plan, and the organization's involvement in external (community-based) and internal drills to practice preparedness for potential disasters. During the development of the disaster preparedness plan, the hospital will assess for potential barriers to its operations (including patient care) during a disaster. The assessment findings and subsequent mitigation factors are incorporated into the disaster preparedness plan during its development. The response phase involves the implementation of the disaster plan during a crisis to provide care, save lives, and restore community health. After the crisis, the recovery phase begins as the community and hospital attempts to establish normal systems of daily operation which could involve repairs to damaged infrastructure, temporary housing, restoration of essential services (eg, transportation, electrical, communication), and health services (eg, primary care, surgical services, mental-health services).[9]

Conceptual model for hospital disaster preparedness

Verheul and Dückers[10] developed a conceptual model for hospital disaster preparation based on definitions of disaster preparation and operationalization in a systematic literature review of 40 articles (**Fig. 1**). The authors define hospital disaster preparedness as follows:

...a capability or capacity to respond to health needs and morbidities disaster-affected populations (external focus) and the ability to stay operational under critical conditions when the demand for care and the availability of time and resources is scarce (internal focus)[10]

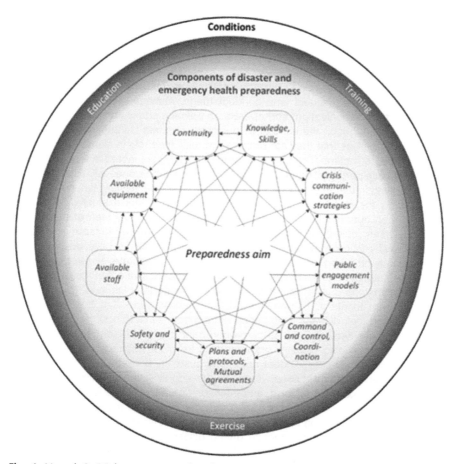

Fig. 1. Vereul & Dückers nonagon for disaster preparedness in hospitals. (Verheul M, Dückers M L A. Defining and operationalizing disaster preparedness in hospitals: A systematic review. Prehosp and Dis Med 2020; 35, 61 – 68.)

At the center of the model is "Preparedness Aim," which is the goal of the organization's efforts concerning disaster preparation. The authors reviewed and organized information from data in the articles describing operationalization of disaster preparation, and then they categorized that information into nine components which they placed in the center of the conceptual model. They assumed that the components are related to each other and that each component must be taken into consideration when developing a disaster response plan. The outer ring of the model depicts the activities that would enhance preparation for disaster planning and assumes that the status of preparedness is dependent on conditions that include education, training, and exercises.[10]

Although the authors indicate the model and its components need further research for clarification and causation between the concepts, a strength of the model is that it identifies the components of disaster preparation. The model factors in the resources of people, equipment, and services, and it identifies the functions of communication, command, and engagement of partners (internal and external), each of which mirrors similar components of the organizational strategic plan familiar to most health care leaders. The conceptual model serves as a guide to health care leaders in the development and review of their organizational disaster preparation plan. Educators can use the model to review curricular components for the education of nursing students on disaster preparedness.

Disaster preparation for nurses

Nurses play a significant role in disasters not only as caretakers for those who are affected but also as rescuers who conduct triage, manage resources, coordinate care, facilitate communication, and operate as trainers, counselors, and information distributors.[9,11] Although the number of declared disasters is increasing worldwide, nurses do not believe that they are prepared to fulfill their role in disasters, including rendering aid to victims.[6,12,13] In one study, researchers noted anecdotally that nursing students participating in a disaster simulation had erroneously assumed staff nurses involved in the project were aware of their facility's disaster plan.[12] In another account from the literature, the authors described an actual explosive event that occurred in an outpatient facility which illuminated the fact that staff at the facility, including nurses, lacked the knowledge and preparation to use the facility's disaster plan.[13] A systematic review of 17 studies revealed that nurses believed they were not adequately prepared for disasters, reporting low-to-moderate levels of preparedness.[14] The authors reported that a majority of nurses were aware that their facility had a disaster plan. One-quarter of nurses had not reviewed the plan, and up to 10% of them could not locate it.[14] Another systematic review supported the finding that nurses believed their disaster preparation ranged from weak to poor.[6]

What do nurses need to know to be prepared for disasters? Common domains of knowledge pertaining to disaster preparedness for nurses include communication, planning, decontamination, incident command systems, and ethics.[9] Labrague and colleagues[14] reported that nurses wanted to develop skills in "first aid training, field triage, advanced basic life support, and infection control."[(p49)] The ICN's Core Competencies in Disaster Nursing Version 2.0 provides additional resources for nursing competency development in disaster preparedness.[8] An additional resource for competency domains for nursing practice during disasters is the ICN's *Core Competencies in Disaster Nursing Version 2.0*.[8] The ICN document provides eight domains with accompanying competencies (**Table 1**) for both the General Professional Nurse and the Advanced or Specialized Nurse. The ICN domains and accompanying competencies comprise a comprehensive, evidence-based competency set that can be

Table 1 International Council of Nurses' domain categories	
Domain	**Category**
1	Preparation and Planning
2	Communication
3	Incident Management
4	Safety and Security
5	Assessment
6	Intervention
7	Recovery
8	Law and Ethics

used by health care organizations as a foundation for training and education of nurses and other staff.[9,14]

Authentic experience in a real disaster is associated with an increase in a nurse's perception of preparedness.[11,14] However, before the COVID-19 pandemic, most nurses reported a lack of experience in actual disaster events. Training coupled with participation in disaster-drill practice also has a positive influence on nurses' belief of preparedness for actual disasters.[13,15,16] The Joint Commission published a standard requiring health care organizations to provide two disaster drills per year for staff training (hospitals may count participation in an actual disaster for one of the drills).[3] Practice drills must be accompanied by other learning methods to introduce nurses to the competencies as outlined by the ICN and the details of organizational disaster plans. Regular practice and ongoing learning are key to maintaining competency and preparedness; modalities of learning include didactic modes, debriefing from events, independent instruction, blended learning, and technology-enhanced learning.[13,15,17,18]

Leaders are challenged to keep their staff ready with an understanding of the disaster plan, preparedness to fulfill their roles in a disaster, and ability to use equipment and protocols that may not be part of their daily routine. This challenge can be met through the use of technology embedded into a preparedness plan. Most staff are familiar with or participate in social media, which is recognized for its educational value.[15] Ghezehjeh and colleagues[15] showed disaster preparedness knowledge in staff nurses, improved with the utilization of social media to deliver training content. Staff nurses received one training per day in the form of text messages, video clips, or images, totaling 34 short training sessions based on disaster preparedness. An educational intervention such as this could augment annual disaster training by providing a steady stream of disaster preparedness content to nurses.

Nursing leaders routinely participate in disaster planning activities. However, staff nurses should have a seat at the table for development, review, and implementation of facility disaster plans. Staff nurses should also be invited to observe their facility Incident Command Center (ICC) in operation. Through observation in the ICC, staff nurses can conceptualize the plan, the role they play within it, and evaluate performance after the event through debriefing.

Disasters can affect any entity, population, and location. They can be external to hospitals (industrial explosions, weather events, transportation accidents, and mass shootings) or be internal as in the example of the explosion at the outpatient facility.[13] Hospitals are additionally vulnerable to disasters. Two examples of disasters that directly impacted hospitals include Hurricane Katrina and the resulting damage to Memorial Medical Center in Houston, Texas, and a tornado that hit St. John's Regional Medical Center in Joplin, Missouri. Internal hospital disasters can take the form of hospital fires, floods, power outages, cyberattacks, or communication and technology failure to name a few.[19] The authors of this article have held leadership roles in a small, community-based, urban hospital and have experienced three declared disasters (one flood and two power outages). The disaster caused by a total hospital power failure, including the backup generator, caused elevators to stop working; stairwells were pitch black; air handlers stopped working, including air conditioning; and computer, phone, and paging systems were all offline. Experiencing a real disaster validates the need for staff nurses to be familiar with how to handle a large-scale crisis in their own environment. Disaster preparation must include training on any contingency plans for computer system or communication failure (including the electronic health record).[19] In a disaster, nurses may find themselves working in unfamiliar settings, unfamiliar circumstances, with unfamiliar equipment, protocols, or other professionals whom they have not worked with before.[2,20] Essential skills such as triage, first aid, evacuation procedures, and knowledge of facility structure (eg, how to close oxygen and other gas lines, location of evacuation routes, and how to use evacuation equipment) should be included in training and reenforced periodically, as with any infrequently used skill. Examples include having all staff, including nurses, complete the Stop the Bleed program for massive hemorrhages or routinely practice using evacuation hammocks in stairwells with mannequins.

Resilience and Mental-Health Interventions

Disasters impact both individuals and groups within a society and can last for brief periods of time to months or years, as with the COVID-19 pandemic.[21] Exposure to such long periods of stress can have a negative impact on the health and well-being of not only the victims of the disaster, but also on those responding as rescuers, including nurses. Such stress reduces the capacity for rescuers to perform and provide care.[21] Building the capacity for resiliency in rescuers is crucial to the mission of responding to disasters. Disaster plans should incorporate resilience and mental-health interventions (short term and long term), not only for the victims, but for rescuers as well.[21] Interventions to increase resiliency can include professional consultations and work structure adjustments. For example, disaster preparedness plans should include on-site chaplaincy, psychological counseling, and the use of telemedicine for long-term needs. Health care leaders should also consider shorter shifts with longer periods of rest for rescuers.[7] Social support is key to helping responders to disasters remain resilient in the face of such stress.[22] However, not all responders will take advantage of mental-health interventions offered to them because of barriers that hinder their use, such as the social stigma associated with mental-health crises.[22] Disaster training curricula should include discussions about psychosocial care, including the topic of social stigma and the role it plays in impeding treatment.

Another source of stress for nurse rescuers is concern for their own family well-being during the disaster and, potentially, the need to inform family members that they will be participating in rescue or care of victims of a disaster.[2] Winans recommends that disaster preparedness includes assisting nurses to preplan with their families for disasters.[20] Nurses may need assistance in talking to their families about the role they will play in a disaster response, and leaders should help nurses structure conversations with their families concerning disaster participation. Decreasing nurses' worry about the safety of their family during a disaster can decrease their distraction during a crisis.

Nurses are one of the first providers to care for disaster victims and can evaluate psychosocial needs that may arise. In a study by Kihc and Simsek,[16] a psychological first-aid training guide was used to educate nursing students. Students who received the training showed an increase in self-efficacy for disaster preparedness compared with the control group. The researchers concluded that the training had a positive effect on self-efficacy for disaster preparedness, including the ability to handle psychosocial issues. Inclusion of psychosocial care for both rescuer and victim should be a standard in disaster training curriculum for nurses.

Disaster preparation for nursing students

Disaster content is not consistently covered in basic nursing education programs, especially in developing countries.[5,12,23] The AACN has endorsed the teaching of disaster preparation and included it in their core competencies for undergraduate and graduate nursing education document titled *The Essentials: Core Competencies for Professional Nursing Education.*[4] Incorporating disaster training into nursing education programs provides an opportunity for nurses in practice to partner with their peers in academia. Such partnerships will support student preparation for clinical practice and achievement of essential clinical skills.

A nurse's participation in disaster drills or an actual disaster increases their confidence to perform successfully in disasters.[5,13,24,25] During drills, students can participate as observers, act as victims, assist with triage, and help with the logistical coordination of the drill itself. When a disaster drill is scheduled, precepted students can observe in the ICC during the drill. Students can participate in mock phone calls, drill discussions, implementation planning, and later, a debriefing of the exercise. Schools of nursing and hospitals are encouraged to make student participation a routine component of drills that are scheduled in advance. Furthermore, nursing faculty members should represent their school of nursing as a participant on the disaster drill planning committee to provide scholarly information (including the latest evidence from the scientific literature), advocate for the school as a resource in actual disasters, aid with student engagement planning, and communicate disaster plan content back to faculty colleagues.

The AACN's Essentials document, or core competencies, states that entry-level professional nurses should be able to "Describe the health and safety hazards of disaster and public health emergencies."[4] The ICN's *Core Competencies in Disaster Nursing Version 2.0* states that a standard professional nurses should meet is "Describes approaches to accommodate vulnerable populations during an emergency or disaster response."[8] One approach to preparing nursing students to achieve these competencies is to develop curricula that engages them with the community. Shannon[26] described a community-based program requiring nursing students to complete a community assessment for disaster preparedness, including a disaster response. In addition, students developed and implemented educational activities for community members on topics of disaster preparation using seminars, social media content, and games.[26] Most hospital systems are required to complete a community assessment as part of their Medicare participation, and nursing students could be valuable partners in this work by assisting with data collection for disaster preparation.

Another teaching strategy to support nursing students' understanding of disaster preparedness is to have them review and analyze a hospital's disaster plan and participate in revising or updating the plan. To gain knowledge of the disaster planning on a macro level, students can use the Nonagon for Disaster Preparedness in Hospitals[10] conceptual model (see **Fig. 1**) to review a hospital's disaster plan. As they delve into the details of the plan, they will learn how each component of the plan works cohesively and identify the resources that will be needed for plan implementation.

Interprofessional education (IPE) in health curricula provides students with opportunities to learn the roles of other professions, practice communication with individuals in other professions, and collaborate during patient care. Establishing disaster drills in a simulation format is one type of IPE that has shown a measure of success.[12,27] Disaster drill simulations are held routinely and often involve hospital participants and local civic organizations (eg, city fire departments, county responders, military units). Nursing student involvement facilitates learning about disaster preparedness, interprofessional communication and collaboration, community resources that are available, and the local community disaster plan. Rotation of roles among participants during a simulation allows everyone to practice various skills with other professions and provides a comprehensive experience.[27]

Educational pedagogies commonly used to prepare nursing students (and practicing nurses) in disaster preparedness include online learning, didactic, independent learning, participation in disaster exercises, and blended learning.[2] Each of these approaches has been successful in increasing self-efficacy for disaster preparedness in students and practicing nurses.[2,13,17,18] A critical feature of disaster preparedness education is practice in application of nursing skills and knowledge in a stressful environment and under less-than-optimal conditions. Simulation has shown consistent success in achieving this goal, and disaster drill simulation exercises provide an experience that has an element of realism for the student to react to.[28,29] Computer software and hardware have advanced to a degree that they serve as effective platforms for disaster preparedness training as well as a useful tools to aid rescuers during an actual disaster event.

Role of technology in disaster preparedness and actual disasters

Nurse educators are challenged to provide engaging education and staff development in safe environments and flexible, accessible formats. Moreover, staff are challenged to find time to participate in educational programs because of critical bedside staffing needs. Incorporating the use of technology to deliver educational programs can resolve some of these challenges, especially when used for disaster preparedness training, as in the example using social media to provide disaster preparation content to emergency department staff nurses.[15] There are many benefits to using relatively simple forms of technology to deliver educational content, such as text messages, including limited human-to-human contact, no need for diverting staff from clinical care, no need for expensive equipment, and minimal overall cost.

More complex learning technologies are used in simulation to teach skills and competencies in disaster preparedness. Simulation is an effective tool for learning because it brings realism to the experience of skill acquisition for the learner, facilitating mastery of competencies under intense, adverse conditions.[30,31] Virtual reality or virtual simulation (VS) is a computer-generated environment in which learners interact with three-dimensional (3D) objects that appear real.[32] VS is used in other industries, including training by the military, aerospace, and airline industries.[17,33] VS offers important benefits to health care educators and leaders, adding value to teaching and learning through facilitation of skill acquisition.[29,32,34,35] Scenarios in VSs can easily be modified to fit educational objectives for a specific audience or skill. Unlike in-person drills that require significant planning, equipment, and funds to prepare and implement, VS scenarios are developed in a virtual world and can be changed more readily through programming. The disaster scenario scalability and complexity can be modified as the participant either gains competency or requires additional practice. In addition, participants can interact in the 3D virtual world through visual, auditory, and tactical senses, further enhancing the learning experience.[18,33] In contrast to live disaster exercises, which are scheduled events usually involving only the staff working on a specific shift, VS exercises allow the greatest number of staff to participate at times convenient for them and their employer.

VS is overall less expensive compared with in-person training. A comparative cost analysis between virtual reality exercises used for disaster preparedness and traditional live exercises showed that cost savings by using VS were significant over time when compared with using live exercises.[34] VS requires significant monetary investment up front with purchase of hardware and software, but this investment is realized over time as the equipment lifespan is 3 to 4 years.[34] As VS technology continues to advance in its sophistication and capabilities, the benefits of VS will continue to overshadow remaining barriers for disaster preparation training. Nurse educators and nursing leaders should develop plans to move disaster preparedness education to the virtual world through VS.

Communication issues pose significant challenges (eg, matching victims needs with responders' resources) to effective disaster response at the time a crisis occurs.[21] In addition, getting information about the disaster itself (eg, reports of washed-out bridges, damaged buildings, power outages, people injured, location of recovery and relief centers) is important for both responders and victims. Leveraging technology through crowdsourcing is one strategy to mitigate these challenges. Crowdsourcing is defined as the use of technology by users to create and curate informational content, collaborating to add and update information primarily on a common communication platform.[36] Guntha and colleagues[37] summarized the positive role crowdsourced communications can play in disaster response to a flood. For example, using a centralized online system accessible to the public, requests for medical assistance, food and water, shelter, transportation, and medicine can be requested by victims through their mobile devices or home computers. Volunteers can access the system to list services, equipment, or supplies being offered. After reviewing all the crowdsourced information, disaster managers can match need with recovery effort. The authors also listed downsides to a crowdsourcing approach to disaster communication, such as disorganization of information, unreliable information, duplicated requests, and hoarding; however, as the technology continues to evolve, solutions to those challenges will likely be resolved over time.[37]

Role of the nurse in technology-based solutions

Nurses have a significant role when technology-based approaches to disaster training and management are used. First, beyond educating themselves on the platforms and contexts where they work best, nurses need to take an active role in educating the public. Nursing students can include information on crowdsourcing systems used in their community as part of their community teaching plans on disaster preparedness. Second, nurses need to know how to use crowdsourcing systems used in their geographical location as they themselves could be a victim of a disaster in their community and may need to use it. Third, health care leaders, including senior nursing leaders, could access the crowdsourcing systems to anticipate both short- and long-term community needs and begin preparations to meet those needs.

As technology continues to advance and become more sophisticated, it offers nurses certain benefits that are essential to preparation for disasters, such as cost-effectiveness, ease of use, mobility, time savings, communication enhancement, and reliability. The nursing discipline will need to embrace the use of technology as a means for safe, effective, low cost, timely education on disaster preparedness. In addition, nurses will need to use technology to manage actual disaster situations both in the short term and long term to plan for and meet the needs of their communities.

Recommendations for Staff Nurse and Nursing Student Disaster Preparation

Disaster events are increasing worldwide, and the nursing profession must be in a state of continual readiness. The following recommendations are offered for nurse leaders and educators to improve readiness for disasters:

- Use a conceptual model (eg, Nonagon for Disaster Preparedness in Hospitals[10]) for hospital disaster plan development and nursing education curriculum development on disaster preparedness.
- Integrate short-term and long-term psychosocial aspects of care for victims and rescuers into disaster plans and education.
- Develop practice-academia partnerships by adding nurse educators to disaster preparedness committees for hospitals.
- Include first-aid training and triage to disaster preparedness education for both nurses and nursing students.
- Embrace a continual readiness approach to education by planning frequent, routine educational activities on the disaster preparedness plan, first aid, and disaster management.
- Involve nursing students in all hospital disaster drill exercises in the roles of both victim and participant.
- Engage students in community education on disaster preparedness.
- Use technology, such as VS, to deliver education on disaster preparedness and provide realistic training for nurses in unfamiliar contexts.
- Encourage community and hospital leaders to explore crowdsourcing technology for potential incorporation into disaster preparedness plans.

SUMMARY

Humanity is facing an increasing threat to life and property due to an increase in disasters.[1–3] Disasters occur with little to no warning and can last hours to months or years. Nursing as a profession must be in a state of constant readiness to render aid as responders to disasters. Leaders must have a mindset of continual readiness and embrace a philosophy of staff and student nurse engagement in disaster plan development, review, and implementation. Educational and training programs should be regular, ongoing, easily accessible, engaging, and based on authentic conditions to deliver education and facilitate communication in actual disasters. The use of technology holds the substantial potential to strengthen disaster preparedness and should be incorporated into disaster preparedness plans.

CLINICS CARE POINTS

- Disaster preparedness programs for staff nurses must contain an element of continuous education.
- Disaster preparedness for staff and nursing students should include basic first aid, triage management, disaster management, and organizational disaster plan content.
- Nursing leaders, faculty, staff, and students are partners in participation during hospital disaster drills and education.
- Nursing faculty and nursing staff should be regular members of hospital disaster preparedness committees.

- Virtual simulation should be embraced as a teaching strategy for disaster preparedness education for nursing students and staff nurses.

DISCLOSURE

The authors have no disclosures regarding the support or work of this article or any of the works cited within. The three authors have no relevant financial or nonfinancial relationships to disclose.

REFERENCES

1. Center for Medicare Services. Emergency preparedness rule. 2016. Available at: https://www.cms.gov/Medicare/Provider-Enrollment-and-Certification/SurveyCertEmergPrep/Emergency-Prep-Rule. Accessed December 28, 2021.
2. Gowing JR, Walker KN, Elmer SL, et al. Disaster preparedness among health professional and support staff: What is effective? An integrative literature review. Prehospital Disaster Med 2017;32:321–8.
3. The Joint Commission. Emergency Management. Available at: https://www.jointcommission.org/resources/patient-safety-topics/emergency-management/. Accessed December 28, 2021.
4. American Association of Colleges of Nursing. The essentials: core competencies for professional nursing education. 2021. Available at: https://www.aacnnursing.org/AACN-Essentials. Accessed December 28, 2021.
5. Kaviani F, Aliakbari F, Sheikhbardsiri H, et al. Nursing students' competency to attend disaster simulations: a study in western Iran. Dis Med and Pub Health Prepard; 2021. https://doi.org/10.1017/dmp.2021.263.
6. Songwathana P, Timalsina R. Disaster preparedness among nurses of developing countries: an integrative review. Internat Emg Nurs 2021;55:2–15.
7. Faccincani R, Pascucci F, Lennquist S. How to surge to face the SARS-CoV-2 outbreak: lessons learned from Lombardy, Italy. Dis Med Pub Health Prepard 2020;14:e39–41.
8. International Council of Nurses. Core competencies in disaster nursing version 2.0. 2019. Available at: https://www.icn.ch/sites/default/files/inline-files/ICN_Disaster-Comp-Report_WEB.pdf. Accessed December 27, 2021.
9. Al Thobaity A, Plummer V, Williams B. What are the most common domains of the core competencies of disaster nursing? A scoping review. Internat Emerg Nurs 2017;31:64–71.
10. Verheul MLMI, Dückers MLA. Defining and operationalizing disaster preparedness in hospitals: a systematic literature review. Prehosp Disaster Med 2020;35:61–8.
11. Taskiran G, Baykal U. Nurses' disaster preparedness and core competencies in Turkey: a descriptive correlational design. Int Nurs Rev 2019;66:165–75.
12. Primeau MS, Benton AM. Multilevel disaster simulation in nursing: Lessons learned in undergraduate and nurse practitioner student collaboration. Nurse Educ Persp 2021;42:188–9.
13. Burnett AL, McGuire K. "This is not a drill – evacuate the building now!" Disaster preparedness at the outpatient surgery department: An experiential lesson. Jour Ped Surg Nurs 2020;9:37–42.
14. Labrague LJ, Hammad K, Gloe DS, et al. Disaster preparedness among nurse: a systematic review of literature. Int Nurs Rev 2017;65:41–53.

15. Ghezeljeh TN, Aliha JM, Haghani H, et al. Effect of education using the virtual social network on knowledge and attitude of emergency nurses of disaster preparedness: A quasi-experimental study. Nurse Educ Today 2019;73:88–93.

16. Kihc N, Simsek N. The effects of psychological first aid training on disaster preparedness perception and self-efficacy. Nurse Educ Today 2019;83:1–8.

17. Duan Y, Zhang J, Xie M, et al. Application of virtual reality technology in disaster medicine. Cur Med Sci 2019;39:690–4.

18. Nguyen VT, Jung K, Dang T. VRescuer: A virtual reality application for disaster response training. 2019. IEEE International Conference on Artificial Intelligence and Virtual Reality. Available at: https://www.researchgate.net/publication/338208720_VRescuer_A_Virtual_Reality_Application_for_Disaster_Response_Training. Accessed December 30, 2021.

19. Barten DG, Klokman VW, Cleff S. When disasters strike the emergency departments: a case series and narrative review. Internat Jour Emerg Med 2021;14:49.

20. Winans M. NICU disaster preparedness: Were we ready for COVID-19? Nurs Leadersh 2020;18:561–4.

21. Hugelius K, Becker J, ADolfsson A. Five challenges when managing mass casualty or disaster situations: a review study. Internat Jour Environ Res Pub Heal 2020;17:1–13.

22. DePierro J, Lowe S, Katz C. Lessons learned from 9/11: mental health perspectives on the COVID-19 pandemic. Psychol Res 2020;288:1–3.

23. Unver V, Basak T, Tastan S. Analysis of the effects of high-fidelity simulation on nursing students' perceptions of their preparedness for disasters. Internat Emerg Nrsg 2018;38:3–9.

24. Gandhi S, Yeager J, Glaman R. Implementation and evaluation of a pandemic simulation exercise among undergraduate public health and nursing students: a mixed-methods study. Nurse Educ Today 2021;98:1–8.

25. Koca B, Arkan G. The effect of the disaster management training program among nursing students. Public Health Nurs 2020;37:769–77.

26. Shannon C. Improving student engagement in community disaster preparedness. Nurse Educ 2019;44:304–7.

27. Innis J, Mack K. Evaluation of nursing students' experience in an interprofessional simulated disaster exercise. Jour Nurse Educ 2021;60:445–8.

28. Caballero AR, Niguidula JD. Disaster risk management and emergency preparedness: a case-driven training simulation using immersive virtual reality. 4th ACM In Cooperation International Conference in HCI and UX 2018. Available at: https://dl.acm.org/doi/abs/10.1145/3205946.3205950. Accessed December 15, 2021.

29. Farra S, Hodgson E, Miller ET, et al. Effects of virtual reality simulation on worker emergency evacuation of neonates. Dis Med Pub Prepar 2018;13:301–8.

30. Harper MG, Bodine J, Monachino A. The effectiveness of simulation use in transition to practice nurse residency programs. Jour Nurs Prof Dev 2021;37:329–40.

31. Dincer B, Ataman H. The effect of high reality simulation on nursing students' knowledge, satisfaction, and self-confidence levels in learning. Intern Jour Car Sci 2020;13:1969–75.

32. Tolarba JEI. Virtual simulation in nursing education: a systematic review. Intern Jour Nurse Educ 2021;13:48–54.

33. Diaz JEM, Saldana CAD, Avila CAR. Virtual world as a resource for hybrid education. Interna Jour Emerg Tech Learn 2020;15:94–109.

34. Farra SL, Gneuhs M, Hodgson E, et al. Comparative cost of virtual reality training and live exercises for training hospital workers for evacuation. Comput Inform Nurs 2019;37:1–16.

35. Shin H, Rim D, Kim H, et al. Educational characteristics of virtual simulation in nursing. An Integr Rev 2019;37:18–28.

36. Huang Y, Sundar SS. Do we trust the crowd? Effects of crowdsourcing on perceived credibility of online health information. Health Commun 2022;37:93–102.

37. Guntha R, Rao SN, Shivdas A. Lessons learned from deploying crowdsources technology for disaster relief during Kerala floods. Proc Comp Sci 2020;171:2410–9.

Nursing Ethics Education
Thinking, Feeling, and Technology

Dónal P. O'Mathúna, PhD

KEYWORDS

- Ethical comportment • Educational technology • Emotions • Microethics
- Macroethics • Motion pictures • Music • Principle-based ethics

KEY POINTS

- Ethics involves thinking and emotions, so ethics education must incorporate strategies that facilitate exploration of the complex, multidimensional aspects of ethics.
- The arts and humanities can bring emotional and relational dimensions of true-to-life scenarios into ethics education to be combined with more philosophic reflection on ethics.
- Technology has an important role in facilitating the exploration of emotional aspects of ethics through film, music, online exhibits, discussion forums and gaming.

BACKGROUND

Technology is increasingly used in nursing education, including in teaching nursing ethics. The coronavirus disease 2019 (COVID-19) pandemic has advanced the move to online education even further. However, empirical investigation into the impact of these changes across health care education has been limited and the findings mixed. For example, an online nursing ethics course held before the pandemic had equivalent positive impacts on the development of ethical competences as a traditional in-person ethics class.[1] An online ethical decision-making framework was used with radiography students to identify and explore ethical values in case scenarios.[2] Focus group interviews were held with 5 students who described the experience positively and said it assisted them to identify their own values and helped them put themselves into others' shoes. A module on ethics in emergency medicine moved to a virtual environment during COVID-19. The students evaluated the course positively, whereas the instructors questioned whether it was equivalent to the usual in-person course involving simulation patients.[3]

Another study developed an interactive situational e-learning system to facilitate ethical decision-making skills in a nursing ethics course.[4] Animated videos were

College of Nursing, and Center for Bioethics and Medical Humanities, The Ohio State University, 1585 Neil Avenue, Columbus, OH 43210, USA
E-mail address: omathuna.6@osu.edu
Twitter: @domathuna (D.P.O.)

Nurs Clin N Am 57 (2022) 613–625
https://doi.org/10.1016/j.cnur.2022.06.009
0029-6465/22/© 2022 Elsevier Inc. All rights reserved.

nursing.theclinics.com

used to present ethical dilemmas to students and provide instruction on an ethics decision-making model. The e-learning system supplemented some sections of the course, whereas other sections received the usual in-person classroom instruction. The nursing students' ethical decision-making competencies were measured before and after each approach using an instrument measuring 6 ethics competencies. Findings showed significant differences between the 2 approaches on only 2 competencies: identifying ethical questions and recognizing differences in values and viewpoints among characters in the scenarios. The investigators pointed to previous research findings that face-to-face discussions may be essential in ethics education. The investigators also cautioned that e-learning systems require more resources to develop, run, and provide support to students and faculty. It was concluded that it was unclear whether the improvements they found in 2 ethics competencies "warrant the extensive effort required to develop and implement e-learning modalities in nursing ethics education."[4(p37)]

THE NATURE OF ETHICS EDUCATION

These examples point to some of the ongoing challenges and questions surrounding the value and limitations of technology in teaching ethics and promoting ethical development. Although ethics is consistently seen as important in nursing, the nature of ethics education and how ethics competencies can be achieved have been debated, with many concerns about how ethics has been taught across health care professions.

Ethics has been at the core of nursing education since its professional development by Florence Nightingale. A 2021 review of the history of nursing in the United Kingdom concluded that Nightingale's legacy in nursing education involved 2 broad areas, "simultaneously nursing science and practice, and moral formation."[5] Moral formation emphasized the development of moral character, which today would be described as a virtue ethics approach. Various character traits or qualities, or virtues, were seen as central to the development and practice of "the good nurse," which always referred to the moral or ethical good. Early nursing literature from the United States regularly discussed "nursing ethics," whereas the UK literature rarely used the term "ethics" but still gave considerable attention to ethical issues.[5] Throughout this article, the words moral, ethical, and their related terms will be used interchangeably.

Although nursing has consistently emphasized ethics, approaches to ethics education have changed within nursing and in other health care professions. The early emphasis on virtue ethics and character formation led to concern in the 1950s around the psychological and intellectual attributes required to be a successful nurse. This concern resulted in reduced emphasis on moral character, and by the 1980s the focus was on duty-based morality, or deontology.[5] A deontological approach to ethics is exemplified by what has been called the four principles approach of Beauchamp and Childress.[6] Their work acknowledges other theoretic approaches to ethics, including virtue ethics and utilitarianism. However, they see the ethical principles of autonomy, beneficence, nonmaleficence, and justice as central to ethical decision making in health care.

The four principles approach has come to characterize bioethics as a discipline;[7] its impact on nursing education can be seen in the definition of ethics in the 2021 American Association of Colleges of Nursing (AACN) core competencies for nursing education entitled *The Essentials.*[8] Having affirmed that ethics is core to professional nursing practice, it states that "ethics refers to principles that guide a person's behavior. Ethics is closely tied to moral philosophy involving the study or examination of morality through a variety of different approaches. There are commonly accepted principles in bioethics that include autonomy, beneficence, non-maleficence, and justice."[8(p13)] *The Essentials* acknowledges ethics concepts like moral distress, moral resilience, and ethical comportment, but emphasizes the application of ethical principles to issues. For example, under population health, the ethics competency for entry-level nursing education is described as identifying "ethical principles to protect the health and safety of diverse populations," and for advanced practice as incorporating "ethical principles in resource allocation in achieving equitable health."[8(p34)] A study of nursing education found that "both students and faculty identified ethics as ethical rights based on the principles of autonomy, beneficence, nonmaleficence, truth telling, just allocation of scarce resources, and fairness."[9(p475)]

Despite the historical and current importance placed on ethics in nursing, nursing ethics faculty in a small qualitative research study reported that ethics content was being pushed aside in nursing curricula because it was viewed as less important than core nursing content.[10] These faculty felt unprepared to teach ethics, with few having any formal education in ethics themselves. The investigators noted that ethical nursing practice requires active engagement in thinking, reasoning, understanding, reflection, and communication, pointing to a similar focus on reasoning skills as seen in *The Essentials*.

Ethical principles and moral philosophy are important in health care ethics, but they are insufficient to promote ethical development. Some studies suggest that nursing ethics courses that focus on ethical principles do not accomplish much learning at all. A small qualitative study of final-semester nursing students explored their ethical decision-making process in a simulated setting.[11] All these students had successfully completed an ethics course that emphasized major ethics theories and their application to health care scenarios, as well as examined ethics case studies in structured and unstructured clinical settings. The researchers found that none of the students deliberately integrated ethical principles during the simulation ethics scenario. The students reported that what they learned in their ethics course had little relevance because it was "philosophical ethics"; as one student stated, "With ethics, it's like you learn it and you forget it."[11(p3)]

Previous research has identified a disconnect between ethical theory and principles and their application in nursing practice. A major study of nursing ethics education found "a tenacious assumption that the students learn abstract information and then apply that information in practice."[12(p14)] Abstract ethical principles are difficult to retain, and students also struggle to see how they apply in clinical practice. "This perceived disconnection between ethics theory and clinical practice, as reported by nurses, may be the reason why nurses tend to demonstrate inconsistent patterns of ethical decision making."[13(p500)]

In addition to an overemphasis on philosophical principles, concerns have been raised about the types of ethics issues addressed in ethics classes. A tendency exists to focus on major ethics issues, like abortion, euthanasia, reproductive technology, and organ transplantation, collectively known as macroethics issues.[11] Although these issues are important, and nursing has a role in each, many ethical issues in nursing practice are less dramatic and more routine. Called *microethics issues*, or *everyday ethics*, they include situations in which colleagues do not follow best practices, disagree over patient safety, and bully each other, and other situations that rarely make headlines but weigh heavily on nurses. Microethics issues are significant and can be the source of substantial confusion, disequilibrium, and moral distress.[14] Nursing scholars have found that with such "multilayered ethical challenges in nursing practice" that "[p]rinciples of bioethics, moral theory and ethical decision-making are not sufficient."[15(p250)]

The type of case studies used in health care ethics education has also been of concern. Case studies are widely valued and commonly used to explore ethical issues. However, a nurse bioethicist and colleagues challenged the way ethics education cases often address macroethics in what they call "tragic cases," not the microethics of everyday practice.[16] Annas[17] has similarly criticized the use of "worst-case scenarios" in planning for public health. The cases in nursing ethics education often examine dilemmas that focus on patients' rights and health care professionals' duties.[9] Cases often are discussed with a view to highlighting clashing values and principles, and how these can be resolved through prioritizing various ethical principles.[18] The problem is that an almost exclusive use of such cases "deludes the student (and subsequent practitioner) into thinking that ethics concerns are rare" when in reality they are part of daily moral experience[16(p674)]; they give the impression that ethics cases should be resolvable once and for all, whereas in reality, many everyday cases are ongoing. Tragic cases can leave students feeling either helpless because they do not know what to do or overly confident that a good decision can always be found. Such cases also suggest that answers are found intellectually and in generalities, whereas real cases are heavily contextualized and involve the views and meanings of several people as well as organizations and society.

A final area of concern with nursing ethics education is an overemphasis on a particular definition of autonomy. A principle-based approach to ethics often leads to a search for the principles in conflict. For example, if a patient refuses to do what a nurse believes is best for him or her autonomy is seen to conflict with beneficence. Given the intractability of such cases, some prioritization of principles is needed. Coupled with the importance of advocacy in nursing, the principle of autonomy has been emphasized in nursing ethics where cases are resolved by identifying which approach best promotes patient autonomy.[18] Such an approach reflects a very narrow view of autonomy, one that conflicts with a relational approach to autonomy.[19] This approach also undermines the need to critically reflect on whether what the patient wants is ethical or not. If the case is resolved by advocating for whatever the patient wants, ethics has been taken out of the deliberations. The difficulties with such a view of autonomy have been clearly seen during COVID-19 as patients, nurses, and others refuse to carry out public health measures that have been deemed to be best for the public good. An exclusively individualized view of autonomy is unworkable in a public health crisis and undermines the possibility of thinking through and evaluating which public health (and individual) measures are most ethical.

ETHICS BEYOND PRINCIPLES

Within ethics, knowledge and understanding of ethical principles and theories are important, but insufficient. The rational side must be accompanied by "recognition and acknowledgment of the centrality of emotions in human relationships."[16(p674)] The role of emotions in ethics is undergoing a significant revival. Throughout the history of philosophy, particularly in moral philosophy, emotions have been ignored or pushed aside as counterproductive for ethics.[20] Important exceptions exist, most notably Aristotle and the eighteenth-century David Hume. At present, research in psychology, anthropology, and other social sciences is renewing interest in the role of emotion, culture, and social factors in ethical decision making.[21] Martha Nussbaum[22] has written extensively on the importance of emotion in ethics. She notes that ethics has been viewed as a system of principles to be grasped in detached ways, with emotions either supporting or subverting our rational choices to act according to principles. Instead, she argues that "emotions are part and parcel of the system of ethical reasoning."[22(p1)] Emotions must be acknowledged and explored, just as reasons and beliefs should be. At the same time, they must be evaluated and not unreflectively accepted as guides to action or given "a privileged place of trust."[22(p1)] Such an approach to ethics has important implications. "We will have to grapple with the messy material of grief and love, anger and fear, and the role these tumultuous experiences play in thought about the good and the just."[22(p1-2)] Research during COVID-19 has shown that nurses' ethical concerns were multiple, complex, and interwoven with many different emotions, including anger, guilt, frustration, and joy.[23]

To include reflection on emotions within ethics, Nussbaum[22] and many others advocate using teaching materials that go beyond standard philosophical texts. Literature, art, music, and film become crucial ways to introduce emotions within everyday ethics; this leads to "making a place for literature (and other works of art) within moral philosophy, alongside more conventional philosophical texts... an account of human reasoning based only upon abstract texts such as are conventional in moral philosophy is likely to prove too simple to offer us the type of self-understanding we need."[22(p3)] Case studies continue to play an important role, but they should promote exploration of the thoughts, feelings, and relationships involved, not just ethical principles. Case discussions should encourage students to explore their thoughts and feelings as they reflect on the case. Ethics cases should look more like stories, where characters, relationships, and cultural factors are developed and explored.

Introducing emotions and stories takes ethics beyond principles, duties, and codes into the arena of virtue ethics. Here, the goal is not only to acquire knowledge of ethics terminology or understand methods to resolve ethical dilemmas. Learning also should include developing ethical traits and characteristics. This approach represents a return to earlier emphases on moral formation of the good nurse: the nurse who knows what is ethical and is motivated to work toward that good, and this must include reflection on the thoughts, beliefs, values, and emotions involved in everyday ethical situations and how these exist and develop in the context of relationships.

ETHICAL COMPORTMENT

Patricia Benner[24] has called for such an approach to ethics, calling it ethical comportment. She holds that becoming a good nurse involves interweaving clinical and ethical reasoning; developing moral imagination, moral agency, and ethical perception skills; and applying these in everyday professional interactions. The AACN *Essentials* defines ethical comportment as, "The way in which nurses embody the ability to relate to others respectfully and responsively."[8(p58)] However, a systematic review of "ethical comportment" included only 20 articles exploring the concept in depth and concluded that even though the term holds "an elevated position in nursing education," it has been marginalized and its development stagnated.[7(p467)] The reviewer speculated that this incongruity may exist because nursing ethics education has been dominated by the principles-based approach to resolving ethical dilemmas that arise from tragic cases.

An understanding of ethical principles and theories is important for ethics competencies, but falls short of the deeply personal, holistic, and relational concept of ethical comportment. Benner and colleagues'[12] research has found that ethical comportment can be developed through experiences and stories wherein nurses (and nursing students) meet the patient as a person, preserve the dignity and personhood of patients, respond to substandard practice in colleagues, advocate for patients, engage in active learning to improve practice individually and collectively, and learn to be present with patients and family in their suffering. The investigators summarize this as "learning to do good nursing practice and to be good nurses."[9(p476)] Interestingly, the only time the word "good" is used in the AACN *Essentials* document is when it refers to "social good."[8(p49)] There is nothing wrong with any of the AACN competencies related to ethics, but they fall short of what ethical comportment means and how it can be attained.

HOW TECHNOLOGY CAN HELP

The challenge is for educators to design ethics education that develops practice-ready nurses who understand what ethical comportment involves (as Benner means), are developing its traits within themselves, and apply the concept in day-to-day patient care. Ethics instruction is underpinned by knowledge, but it is fulfilled by shaping attitudes. Technology provides both challenges and opportunities for teaching nursing ethics in alignment with the development of ethical comportment. Technology allows for the ready introduction of various media that explore the emotional, spiritual, relational, and cultural dimensions of ethics. However, technology has the potential to become impersonal, especially when authentic in-person contact and interaction becomes limited. While acknowledging such limitations and challenges, several technology-supported instructional approaches can be used to bring emotional and relational elements into ethics education.

Case Studies

The selection of case studies and how they are discussed is guided by educators' underlying approach to ethics education. Case studies can focus on a clash between ethical principles that can be resolved in rational ways, or they can go deeper into the messiness and discomfort of real life, which can also have moments of joy and connection. Case studies that incorporate the complex emotional realities of clinical situations are available, such as ones exploring whether to visit a dying mother during COVID-19 and risk bringing the virus home to an at-risk husband,[25] how to interact with a mentally disabled man,[26] or whether to give water orally to a boy with traumatic brain injury.[27]

Each of these cases could be explored to identify clashing ethical principles. Instead, the authors introduced an important turn into their narratives. The daughter deciding whether to visit her mother read Nussbaum and allowed her emotions into her considerations. "Bringing emotion into the theoretical frame means that subjectivity, gut feelings, and kinship and friendship ties can be embraced and theorised rather than rejected as 'murky contaminants to reason'," she wrote.[25(p2645)] This did not decide the matter but helped her go beyond the "hollowness" of moral theories and principles, leading to a better way to decide. Another case examined an ethics consultation regarding resource allocation decisions for a 21-year-old man with severe mental retardation.[26] The discussion stalled over which ethical principles and duties were more applicable until the ethicist asked the clinicians some different questions, like "what was this patient like?" and "How do you feel about him?"[26(p280)] Those questions opened completely different conversations that led to agreement on the best way forward. The third example case involved a 6-year-old boy, kicked in the head by a mule. The ethical dilemma was whether to give him fluids or food orally. The situation seemed like "a lost cause" until the nurse took a different view. "I looked at him and felt for the first time since I'd been caring for him that he was looking at me—not the vacant, wild-eyed look I'd grown accustomed to, but an understanding, 'with-it' gaze I had not seen before."[27(p5)] Remembering an order allowing oral fluids, the nurse gave the boy some water, which he gulped down. In this case, the nurse reflected on how she had dismissed the boy's parents because they were quiet and relied on prayer, while she had labeled the boy in a way that dulled "good nursing sense."[27(p7)] Such honesty and humility help to make case reflections more realistic.

Instead of staying at the level of ethics principles and straightforward resolutions, the authors went deeper, usually by asking questions about the emotions or relationships involved. This approach allowed a fuller analysis of the scenarios that led to more authentic and personal ethics discussions. The way these cases are discussed and explored points to the importance of how ethics discussions are facilitated. As cases that focus only on ethical principles are incomplete, so too are stories that only release emotions and leave them poured out on the classroom floor (or the online platform). The facilitator has a vital role in selecting items and asking carefully considered questions at the right time; this is because "it is not all about emotions, since emotions alone are not enough for providing experiences through reflection. The emotional impact caused by emotions should be utilized to foster reflection and this experience generates possibilities for incorporating stable attitudes."[28(p78)]

Film

Technology allows the use of ethics cases from other media. Film has long been seen as having the power to engage people in all parts of their being: emotionally, cognitively, relationally, and morally.[29] Film clips are particularly helpful in bringing emotions into discussions and encouraging reflective learning.[28] One movie distribution company, Movies Change People, selects movies that "stir the spirit" through real-life "messy stories" that address the ethical complexities of issues like poverty, homelessness, suicide, inequity, and others.[30] An integrative literature revealed that films in nursing ethics education can promote student-centered learning, experiential learning, reflective learning, and problem-solving learning.[31] However, the films, or clips from them, must be carefully selected to ensure they match the learning objectives for the class or topic. For example, television (TV) medical dramas often include case studies that revolve around ethical issues. However, such dramas regularly portray medical details inaccurately. For example, a review of more than 200 episodes of TV dramas showing cardiopulmonary resuscitation (CPR) found that the techniques were "mostly portrayed inaccurately."[32(p238)] Consistently, the success rate of CPR in TV dramas is much higher than in reality, which has implications for ethical decision making. At the same time, a growing number of resources are available to identify films and clips that accurately engage with ethical issues and can be incorporated easily into ethics classes whether virtual or in person (**Table 1**).

In choosing films and clips, decisions must also be made about whether to portray dramatic, tragic cases or explore everyday ethics. A movie like *Wit* powerfully displays the everyday interactions between a patient and her health care professionals.[33] The original script was written for the stage, and the patient speaks to the camera to reveal her inner thoughts and feelings about her cancer diagnosis, throwing up after chemotherapy, and the continual clinical concern to measure her various inputs and outputs. These are the everyday practices that engage nurses and come to the fore when they must decide whether to routinely measure urinary output or sit with the patient for a few minutes to talk about how they are feeling and coping. *Wit* also has intense scenes around macroethics issues, such as when a nurse refuses to allow a doctor to perform CPR on a patient with a do-not-resuscitate order, but most of the scenes explore the smaller everyday decisions that are part of ethical comportment.

Songs

Music has been used in moral education since at least the ancient Greeks. Songs with lyrics have an added advantage when they explicitly explore ethical issues. Students

Table 1
Teaching strategies and resources for ethics education

Teaching Strategy	Role in Ethics Education	Educational Resources (Exemplars)	References
Case studies	Permit the exploration of ethical issues in specific scenarios. Cases range from thin descriptions focused on ethical principles to thicker stories engaging characters holistically Discussions can be enhanced using student response systems (eg, Nearpod, Poll Everywhere)	Nursing Case Studies (https://nursingcasestudies.com/) Practical Bioethics resources (https://www.practicalbioethics.org/resources/) World Health Organization, *Ethics in epidemics, emergencies and disasters* (https://www.who.int/publications/i/item/ethics-in-epidemics-emergencies-and-disasters-research-surveillance-and-patient-care-training-manual) Branching scenarios, eg, H5P (https://h5p.org/branching-scenario)	16,25–27
Film	Engages students emotionally, cognitively, relationally, and ethically	Teach with Movies (https://teachwithmovies.org/moral-ethical-emphasis-index/) UNHCR and refugees (https://www.unhcr.org/innovation/7-videos-guaranteed-to-change-the-way-you-see-refugees/) YouTube	29,30
Literature	Portrays fuller development of character, relationships, and affective dimensions of ethics	Numerous, eg, American Library Association list, Ethics through Literature (https://www.ala.org/aboutala/offices/resources/ethics)	22
Songs	Lyrics can explore ethical issues with music triggering emotions in a nonthreatening way	Spinditty playlists (https://spinditty.com/) Experience: Ethics and Equity playlist (https://expmag.com/2020/12/the-experience-playlist-ethics-and-equity/)	34,35
Art	Explore how to handle emotions depicted in art such as anger, compassion, or joy	AMA Journal of Ethics Art Gallery (https://journalofethics.ama-assn.org/art-gallery) National Gallery of Art (https://www.nga.gov/) Jon Lezinsky (https://jonlezinsky.com/) Twitter (especially during COVID-19)	

	Description	Resources/Examples	
Photographs	Capture the emotional and relational dimensions associated with ethical issues	World Health Organization Photo Gallery (https://photos.hq.who.int/) Desperate Journey, *Time* (https://time.com/rohingya-exodus-myanmar-refugees-kevin-frayer/)	
Discussions	Allow students to share their ethics views, explore with others, critically reflect and interact, and engage socially	Integrated into learning management system discussion tools (eg, Canvas, Blackboard) Video- and audio-supported discussion tools available (eg, Flipgrid, VoiceThread)	36-38
Game-based learning	Can allow more realistic exploration of ethics through participation in games and simulations. May allow affective and cognitive learning but requires more resources and guidance	*Games and Ethics*, Springer, 2020 (https://link.springer.com/book/10.1007/978-3-658-28175-5) Nearpod (https://nearpod.com/) Kahoot! (https://kahoot.com/)	39,40

readily engage with the stories contemporary songs tell.[34] Songs can be used to illustrate ethics theories and concepts[35]; they can also go much deeper. Carefully crafted songs use their musical elements to trigger emotions, which then reinforce the messages conveyed through the lyrics. Songs have been cataloged according to their themes to facilitate selection (see **Table 1**). Many contemporary musicians make their songs freely available, particularly through online music platforms. Using songs in ethics education requires asking questions about the words, thoughts, and feelings communicated, and encouraging careful reflection on the messages received. Nursing students have reported that contemporary songs in ethics courses helped them think more deeply about ethics situations and issues in a nonthreatening way.[34]

Art

Technology can make works of art available that otherwise would have required visiting museums, galleries, or other institutions. Many such organizations are making their resources available online (see **Table 1** for sources of the items mentioned in this paragraph). Photographs are readily available online and trigger emotional reactions when they depict topics related to ethics; these can include anger at injustice, compassion from seeing pain and suffering, or joy at moral courage or overcoming challenges. During COVID-19, online art was used to express the complex emotions of health care workers. Use of online photographs and other works of art in ethics education requires careful attention to the images and items selected because teachers will likely not be present to monitor students' reactions when they view them.

DISCUSSION

Face-to-face classroom discussions are highly valued in ethics education, and some view them as essential.[4] However, online discussions can have important advantages, even those that are text based. Evaluations of online discussions found that some students felt greater freedom to share their thoughts and emotions in online settings.[3] Asynchronous online discussion forums can promote self-awareness and self-knowledge (important for ethical awareness) as well as critical reflection.[36] Well-designed asynchronous discussions can help quieter students express their ideas and actively engage with learning, but can feel like a tedious, meaningless chore for students and instructors when not designed well or overused.[37] A review of research in this area found that the format of the tasks given to the students, and how instructors engage in the discussions, strongly influenced student learning. This review also found that cognitive and affective domains need to be addressed in asynchronous discussions, although little research has been conducted in this area. The investigator provided a detailed list of teaching strategies to promote effective learning.[36]

Online discussions can use technology to go beyond text-based discussions through Web-based videoconferencing platforms (like Zoom or Teams). These platforms allow some of the advantages of face-to-face conversations even when students are not together. Students can be divided into small groups to promote learning that includes social presence and group dynamics.[37] The video component can have drawbacks, such as when students have strong beliefs about not being photographed or are very concerned about their appearance. Video discussions may happen synchronously, or the technology can be used asynchronously by encouraging the use of audio or video clips in asynchronous posts or other assignments.[38] For example, students could be asked to record some of their discussion posts rather than putting them into text, or to give recorded presentations as assignments. Many other practical suggestions for using technology in online ethics education have been published, including game-based learning,[39] simulation-based learning, learning through forums, and collaborative digital learning (see **Table 1**).[40]

SUMMARY

Online technology brings many opportunities for ethics education. Virtual learning environments lack some physical classroom features, where teachers can do in-person monitoring of a discussion or exploration of a case study or film clip. For example, additional information can be released as discussions develop, or carefully crafted questions can be asked at opportune times to take the discussion into a deeper or different direction. Students who may not be "getting it" can be more easily identified in person, as can others who may be overwhelmed by emotions or reliving difficult experiences in their own lives. Body language and tone of voice are important elements of in-person discussions, particularly on challenging topics. Online environments, especially asynchronous courses, raise challenges in these areas. At the same time, animated videos, escape rooms, and educational games can be developed or adapted for virtual learning environments to facilitate technology-based discussions. As with any strategy, time must be invested in understanding the strengths and limitations of technology-supported ethics education and ensuring it is molded to the specific learning objectives and context. This fact points to the importance of online educators having the training, technological support, and resources available to adapt their teaching strategies to technology-based learning.

Ethics education is increasingly being examined to determine whether it helps people become more ethical and better prepared to address ethics in the real world. A focus on the cognitive and knowledge dimensions of ethics is insufficient to prepare nurses for the broader dimensions of ethical comportment and related concepts, which require engaging with the affective, personal, and relational dimensions of ethics. Doing so can not only be more challenging, especially in an online environment, but also more engaging and satisfying. More evaluation of the effectiveness of various teaching strategies is important if we are to prepare nurses and other health care professionals to better address the everyday ethics of practice and explore the emotional dimensions of ethics.

CLINICS CARE POINTS

- Ethical principles and theories in ethics education are important, but they must be accompanied by exploration of emotions, culture, and social factors in ethical decision making.

- Traditional ethics education tends to focus on macroethics (broad ethical issues and dramatic cases), but students also need to explore microethics, involving everyday issues of ethical comportment in nursing practice.

- Ethics case studies in nursing education should cover contextualized, real-world situations that involve multiple perspectives and explore cognitive and affective aspects of scenarios lacking ideal resolutions.

- Technology can support ethics education for nurses through film, art, music, online discussions, and simulations.

- Faculty development and support in design and delivery of technology-facilitated ethics education helps ensure nursing ethics competencies can be achieved.

DISCLOSURE

The author has nothing to disclose.

REFERENCES

1. Trobec I, Starcic AI. Developing nursing ethical competences online versus in the traditional classroom. Nurs Ethics 2015;22(3):352–66.
2. Mc Inerney J, Lees A. Values exchange: using online technology to raise awareness of values and ethics in radiography education. J Med Rad Sci 2018;65(1): 13–21.
3. Gintrowicz R, Pawloy K, Richter J, et al. Can we adequately teach ethics and ethical decision making via distant learning? A pandemic pilot. GMS J Med Educ 2020;37(7):Doc80.
4. Chao SY, Chang YC, Yang SC, et al. Development, implementation, and effects of an integrated web-based teaching model in a nursing ethics course. Nurse Educ Today 2017;55:31–7.
5. Fowler MD. The nightingale still sings: ten ethical themes in early nursing in the United Kingdom, 1888-1989. J Issues Nurs 2021;26:2.
6. Beauchamp TL, Childress JF. Principles of biomedical ethics. 8th edition. New York: Oxford University Press; 2022.
7. Hardin J. Everyday ethical comportment: an evolutionary concept analysis. J Nurs Educ 2018;57(8):460–8.
8. American Association of Colleges of Nursing (AACN). The essentials: core competencies for professional nursing education. 2021. Available at: https://www.aacnnursing.org/AACN-Essentials. Accessed February 27, 2022.
9. Benner P, Sutphen M, Leonard-Kahn V, et al. Formation and everyday ethical comportment. Am J Crit Care 2008;17:473–6.
10. Grason S. Teaching ethics in classroom settings: nursing faculty perceptions in baccalaureate programs. J Nurs Educ 2020;59(9):506–9.
11. Krautscheid LC, Brown M. Micro-ethical decision making among baccalaureate nursing students: a qualitative investigation. Faculty Publications - College of Nursing; 2014. Available at: https://digitalcommons.georgefox.edu/sn_fac/31. Accessed February 27, 2022.
12. Benner P, Sutphen M, Leonard-Kahn V, et al. Educating nurses: a call for radical transformation. San Francisco (CA): Jossey Bass; 2010.
13. Callister LC, Luthy KE, Thompson P, et al. Ethical reasoning in baccalaureate nursing students. Nurs Ethics 2009;16:499–510.
14. Gallagher A. Moral distress and moral courage in everyday nursing practice. Online J Issues Nurs 2010;16:2.
15. Doane G, Pauly B, Brown H, et al. Exploring the heart of ethical nursing practice: implications for ethics in education. Nurs Ethics 2004;11:240–53.
16. Liaschenko J, Oguz NY, Brunnquell D. Critique of the "tragic case" method in ethics education. J Med Ethics 2006;32:672–7.
17. Annas GJ. Worst case bioethics: death, disasters, and public health. Oxford: Oxford University Press; 2010.
18. Edwards S. A principle-based approach to nursing ethics. In: Davis S, Tschudin V, de Raeve L, editors. Essentials of teaching and learning in nursing ethics : perspectives and methods. London: Churchill Livingston; 2006. p. 55–66.
19. Greaney A-M, O'Mathúna DP, Scott PA. Autonomy and choice in healthcare: self-testing devices as a case in point. Med Health Care Philos 2012;15(4):383–95.

20. Molewijk B, Kleinlugtenbelt D, Widdershoven G. The role of emotions in moral case deliberation: theory, practice, and methodology. Bioethics 2011;25(7):383–93.
21. Haidt J. The emotional dog and its rational tail: a social intuitionist approach to moral judgment. Psychol Rev 2001;108(4):814–34.
22. Nussbaum MC. Upheavals of thought: the intelligence of emotions. Cambridge: Cambridge University Press; 2001.
23. Kelley MM, Zadvinskis IM, Miller PS, et al. United States nurses' experiences during the COVID-19 pandemic: a grounded theory. J Clin Nurs 2021;31(15–16):2167–80. Online ahead of print.
24. Benner P. Honoring the good behind rights and justice in healthcare when more than justice is needed. Am J Crit Care 2005;14:152–6.
25. Greenhalgh T. Moral uncertainty: a case study of Covid-19. Patient Educ Couns 2021;104(11):2643–7.
26. Reich WT. Caring for life in the first of it: moral paradigms for perinatal and neonatal ethics. Semin Perinatol 1987;11(3):279–87.
27. Benner P. The role of experience, narrative, and community in skilled ethical comportment. Adv Nurs Sci 1991;14(2):1–21.
28. Blasco PG, Moreto G, Pessini L. Using movie clips to promote reflective practice: a creative approach for teaching ethics. Asian Bioeth Rev 2018;10:75–85.
29. Shapshay S, editor. Bioethics at the movies. Baltimore (MD): Johns Hopkins University Press; 2009.
30. Movies Change People. Available at: https://www.movieschangepeople.com/. Accessed February 27, 2022.
31. McAllister M, Levett-Jones T, Petrini MA, et al. The viewing room: a lens for developing ethical comportment. Nurse Educ Pract 2016;16:119–24.
32. Ramirez L, Diaz J, Alshami A, et al. Cardiopulmonary resuscitation in television medical dramas: results of the TVMD2 study. Am J Emerg Med 2021;43:238–42.
33. McConnell T. She's DNR!" "She's research!": conflicting role-related obligations. In: Shapshay S, editor. Bioethics at the movies. Baltimore: Johns Hopkins University Press; 2009. p. 186–201.
34. O'Mathúna DP. Teaching ethics using popular songs: feeling and thinking. Monash Bioeth Rev 2008;27(1–2):42–55.
35. Mizzoni J. Teaching moral philosophy with popular music. Teach Ethics 2006;6(2):15–28.
36. Donlan P. Use of the online discussion board in health professions education: contributions, challenges, and considerations. J Contin Educ Health Prof 2019;39(2):124–9.
37. Serembus JF, Murphy J. Creating an engaging learning environment through video discussions. Nurse Educ 2020;45(2):68–70.
38. Reyes I, Clement D, Sheridan T, et al. Connecting with students: using audio-enhanced discussion boards in a nursing curriculum. Nurse Educ 2020;45(2):71–2.
39. Katsarov J, Biller-Andorno N, Eichinger T, et al. uMed: your choice - conception of a digital game to enhance medical ethics training. In: Groen M, Kiel N, Tillmann A, et al, editors. Games and ethics: theoretical and empirical approaches to ethical questions in digital game cultures. Wiesbaden: Springer; 2020. p. 197–212.
40. Michl S, Katsarov J, Krug H, et al. Ethics in times of physical distancing: virtual training of ethical competences. GMS J Med Educ 2021;38:1.

Future Perspectives on Nursing Policy, Technology, Education, and Practice

Sunny Biddle Nethers, MSN, RN[a,b,*], Jeri A. Milstead, PhD, RN[c]

KEYWORDS

- Nursing education • Information science • Public policy • Health care

KEY POINTS

- Governmental laws and regulation affect nurse practice at the point of care.
- Public and private sector health-care agency policies direct the use of technology in the agency.
- A strong focus on the process of policy making in the nurse education curricula prepares nurses to make sustainable change for the profession and be effective leaders in the boardroom.
- Creating, implementing, and evaluating policies is an integral part of basic and advanced nurse practice.
- Emerging issues of policy, technology, education, and practice must be considered part of the nurse leadership role.

INTRODUCTION

Nursing practice today encompasses many roles in many settings. Most twentieth-century nurses practiced in a hospital but that is changing. Today, nurses have important roles in schools, clinics, long-term care, industry, and a variety of other contexts. The COVID-19 pandemic has demonstrated that public health is in need of modernization to keep the global population healthy, and nurse educators are examining how they can prepare nurses for this decade and beyond. The nurse role has expanded beyond hospitals to schools, clinics, and communities, and practitioners must be prepared as leaders in the art and science of what Nightingale envisioned for the profession: critical thinking, involvement in public policy (not just legislation), global perspectives, and the delicate intersection between personal rights and public good.[1] Educators must make clear the link between practice and policy.

a Central Ohio Technical College Nursing Faculty, 15555 Mary Ann Furnace Road, Newark, OH 43055, USA; b Genesis Healthcare System, 2951 Maple Avenue, Zanesville, OH 43701, USA; c 3170 Kingstree Court, Dublin, OH 43017, USA
* Corresponding author. Genesis Healthcare System, 2951 Maple Avenue, Zanesville, OH 43701, USA
E-mail address: nethers.62@mail.cotc.edu

Nurs Clin N Am 57 (2022) 627–638
https://doi.org/10.1016/j.cnur.2022.06.010
0029-6465/22/© 2022 Elsevier Inc. All rights reserved.

What Is Policy?

Public policy process

The public process of policy making, in simple terms, is identifying a health issue or problem, bringing it to the attention of government, and obtaining a response. Components of the process include agenda setting, government response, and designing, implementing, and evaluating the policy or program. The policy-making process is not linear, and a nurse may enter the process at any point. The *agenda* is a list of items to which the president or governor pays attention and allocates significant funding. Government response usually occurs through legislators in the form of a law, regulation (also known as a rule), or program. Nurses are innovators with pragmatic experience who have valuable roles in designing programs and establishing eligibility criteria for participation. Implementation involves choosing which bureau will house a program (ie, determine which agency has adequate staff, expertise, and commitment to carry out the legislative intent). Evaluation entails gathering appropriate data to determine the relative success of a program. Nurses have many opportunities to work with and guide legislators, agency directors, and staff throughout the policy-making process.

For example, information technology (IT) policies must ensure that government-based regulations such as HIPAA are being followed.[2] Historically, evidence-based policies were not used to address how technology was used in health care. Today, health IT is a continuously dynamic entity, which means that health-care organizations need to evaluate and update policies continually. Many technologies facilitate provision of health care such as portable cellular devices, email, Bluetooth devices, tablets, smart watches, or telehealth visits via institution-owned and patients' personal devices. Technology changes rapidly with new iterations of old equipment or completely new devices to assist caregivers. Nurses have many opportunities to guide legislators through the policy-making process by becoming their expert contacts to educate and clarify health issues.

Private sector policy

Policies are a set of directives that guide the decision-making process of an organization, given a set of specific circumstances. The term *policy* is often accompanied by the term *procedure*; nursing procedures are task-focused and will not be discussed within the context of this article. Policies reflect the philosophy and beliefs of an administration and can be found within the mission, vision, and values statements of the organization. For example, policies found in a Mormon, Jewish, or Catholic health-care agency would reflect a corresponding belief system. Policies are strategic in that they reflect the long-term goals of an organization. Short-term policies often govern the day-to-day operations of staff and communicate expectations for the employees. These policies may be specific to a department (such as nursing or medicine) and are generally based on established standards of practice or evidence-based research conducted within the profession. Each organization must develop its own set of policies that reflect the standards of practice set forth by governing bodies and adhere to governmental laws and regulations. Dissemination can come in the form of in-house notices or memos, online continuing education (CE), email, review in daily huddles, or even bathroom reading material. Nurses must learn how to work in the policy arena to fulfill our role as professionals and leaders. Nursing is regulated by state and federal laws and rules that influence our practice from the bedside to the boardroom.

Governmental and Nongovernmental Organizations

Boards of nursing

A board of nursing is the legal, governmental agency that interprets and promulgates laws and regulations (rules) regarding nursing. Each state and jurisdiction (eg, US territory) has a Boards of nursing (BON) created by the relevant legislative body. BON members are appointed by the governor, except for North Carolina (NC) where 11 of 14 nurse members are elected by all licensed NC nurses. BONs are committed to the protection of the public through the regulation of nursing practice, as opposed to professional associations that serve and promote the interests of member nurses. In their regulatory practice, BON rules have the power of law. Nurses have an opportunity to serve on a BON but must realize that appointment is a political process and, therefore, intentionally develop a path to a leadership role on a BON (see "Toolkit of policy resources" section below). Nurses can also seek appointment, usually by the BON itself, to board committees that address specific issues such as practice and education.

The Nurse Practice Act

The Nurse Practice Act (NPA) is the common term for the collection of regulations known as the administrative code. NPAs traditionally include criteria and composition of a board and relevant committees, definitions, and scope of practice of nurses (Registered nurses (RNs), Licensed practical nurses (LPNs)/Licensed vocational nurses (LVNs)) and others within its purview, license requirements (eg, term, relicensure, disciplinary action, processes), and requirements for nurse education programs (eg, criteria for administrators and faculty, required program content). BONs mostly have jurisdiction over prelicensure programs but may be involved in acknowledgment or regulation of advanced practice. Rules may specify license fees and academic requirements such as the proportions of time required in class, laboratory, and clinical settings. Recently, BONs have directed rules about the extent of the use of simulation as a laboratory tool or a substitute for direct clinical experience.

Nurses have an opportunity to provide input regarding changes in regulations through a process in which BONs review all rules on a regular basis. This process is considered part of a "sunshine" approach to government in which transparency is evident to all citizens. Often, BONs will assess rules in "batches" (ie, a few sessions each year for a specified period until all rules have been reviewed). Board meetings follow a formal process in which nonboard members must seek prior approval to speak during a session for a limited time. A board may set up "interested party" (IP) meetings in which a specific batch of rules or other relevant business is discussed in an informal session open to all nurse input. Nurses should watch for meeting announcements and take the opportunity to participate in discussions and make suggestions for change (**Box 1**).

National Council of State Boards of Nursing

National Council of State Boards of Nursing (NCSBN) is a quasi-governmental, voluntary, independent organization of state or jurisdictional BONs. NCSBN develops and

---

Box 1
Example of a change in a rule

During review of a batch of rules by a BON, a nurse discovered that required curricular content included material from natural sciences, social sciences, and nursing science—but not from the humanities. She wrote a one-page letter to the Assistant Attorney General (counsel for the BON) notifying intent to attend the IP meeting to discuss the inclusion of the humanities in the rule. Her rationale-included recognition that ethics is not learned by studying anatomy and physiology, and social justice is not learned by studying the Krebs cycle—these concepts (crucial to nursing) are drawn from the humanities. The board accepted the nurse's request.

directs the administration of a National Council Licensing Exam for Registered Nurse and Practical/Vocational Nurse. This organization sets the pass rate for BONs.

Telehealth has enhanced opportunities to provide nursing care remotely because it allows a nurse in one state or facility to care for a patient in another. During the past several years, NCSBN has developed a multistate license known as the Nurse Licensure Compact (NLC or Compact). Guided by an Interstate Commission of Nurse Licensure Compact Administrators (ICNLCA), this license "enhances mobility and public protection through maintaining uniform license standards among party state boards of nursing; promoting cooperation and collaboration between party states, facilitating exchange of data and information between party states, and educating stakeholders."[3] By the end of 2021, 38 BONs were participating. Nonparticipating BONs questioned several segments of the Compact, for example, discipline. If a nurse is disciplined by one state, how are other states notified, and is there a continuation of the disciplinary action within the other states? Another issue is whether the ICNLCA usurps the authority of the home BON. Nurses must familiarize themselves with perceived barriers and opportunities that the NLC provides in care delivered across state lines through advances in technology.

Other governmental agencies

Some governmental agencies that do not seem to be related to health issues do, in fact, influence policy. For example, the Department of Veterans Affairs (VA) is focused on individuals who have served in the military. However, the VA has a history of designing, implementing, and evaluating pilot projects related to health care. The VA was an early adopter of electronic health records. Private sector organizations benefitted from the advantages and barriers that were discovered as the VA often served as sites for demonstration projects in which new ideas for health care were tested. The US Department of Transportation (DOT) deals with many issues directly and indirectly related to health care. The DOT has developed a Transportation and Health Tool (THT) with the Centers for Disease Control and Prevention that tracks air quality in major US cities. Motor vehicle crashes are a leading cause of death, and THT collects data and advocates for alternative conveyances and improved roadways. Data also compare benefits and burdens of neighborhoods known to have concentrations of vulnerable populations. These data are used by city planners in recognizing and addressing inequities such as housing affordability, need for improved pedestrian infrastructure, and unaffordable fees for public transportation.[4]

Nongovernmental agencies

Nongovernmental agencies (also known as private sector agencies) such as hospitals, long-term care facilities, and rehabilitation centers must comply with legal rules but also enact their own policies and procedures. Although this article focuses on public policy, the nurse can extrapolate parts of the process to the private sector. What are your organization's policies regarding the use of technology? Do you know where to find those policies? Do you know the process of changing policy within your organization? How can you have an impact on your organization's policies or be part of the change process? How do you get involved in the policy process? These are all questions that nurses must ask to understand the rules and regulations and recommend change for continuous improvement in the organization.

Changing policies in the private sector

The process of changing policies in any organization takes time, research, education, and evaluation. Whether updating old policies or implementing new policies, the process remains relatively similar. Every policy change process must have certain key elements. The first step in policy change is recognizing there is a need for change and putting together a committee to discuss the issue and lead the charge. Often, the nurse is the team member who recognizes that policies are outdated, or new policies are needed. Policy makers are more likely to listen to groups rather than to individuals. Many organizations convene task forces or committees to review, revise, and create new policies. Committees can consist of a variety of members within the organization such as physicians, nurses, patient care technicians, and any additional stakeholders who may be affected by the change. Once a committee has been formed, members research the issue in several ways. For example, they may find out what other (or affiliated) organizations are doing, review the literature, or complete site visits to gain information. Seeking the opinions of a variety of stakeholders builds a coalition that can move an issue up in priority on a policy maker's agenda. Committees gather information by way of anonymous surveys, open forums, and comment boxes.[5] A draft of the new and revised policies should be drawn up and distributed to those who are affected directly and indirectly.

Changing policy in the public sector
The massive bureaucracy of federal and state government may seem intimidating to nurses who are not educated in governmental affairs. If a nurse focuses on one segment of one policy or program in one department or bureau, change becomes more attainable. Nurses need to know where they can find information about the status of any policy. Budget figures, evaluation reports, and media announcements are a few places one can gather information and data. The Federal Register[6] announces new government policies and presents notices of amending and revising current policies. The Federal Register invites comments from the public in oral and written form and must consider all comments during the process of making change. This is an ideal place for nurses to use their voices to influence policy.

Policy evaluation in the public sector
With any policy change, there needs to be a way to evaluate the change in both the short and long terms. Evaluation of a policy determines if the policy was effective (did it have the intended impact?), efficient (did it reach the expected number of people?), and whether it needs revision. Indicators are measurable benchmarks used to determine if a change is achieving the desired outcomes.[7] Indicators should be reviewed and updated throughout the term of the policy change to ensure continued strength of outcomes.[8] Formal evaluators may be appointed or hired to conduct an evaluation of a program. An interim report may be distributed to agency directors to share the findings and direction to date. A final report is provided to the director who makes decisions about whether to make changes.

Relevance of the Public Policy Process to Nurse Education

Integral or add-on?
Policy education is integrated into nurse curricula in quantity and quality that varies widely from one nursing program to another. Most programs introduce the legislative process in undergraduate courses but focus on how a bill becomes a law and not on the broader process of policy making. Graduate programs may have stand-alone policy courses or integrate policy content into other courses. The American Association of Colleges of Nursing (AACN)[9] designated policy as a thread to be woven throughout curricula rather than 1 of the 10 focal content areas that must be included in every nurse curriculum. When the AACN created the "Essentials: Core Competencies for Professional Nurse Education,"[9] they argued that policy should be a thread rather than a major content domain in nurse curricula because, in part, not enough faculty

are knowledgeable or experienced enough to teach the content. Dr Jeri Milstead (written communication January 2020) argued, along with others who thought policy should be elevated to a domain in the Essentials, that there is a block of content that is critical for understanding the process and the need for nurse involvement. Understanding the process of decision-making in a policy setting is crucial to the well-being and future of nursing, health care, and the global economy. The essential question is: To what extent should nurses be knowledgeable and involved in health policy, and where will nurses learn about it? **Box 2** proposes potential solutions to providing policy content throughout the curriculum.

De Cordova and colleagues[10(p44)] wrote "The current healthcare environment is ready for graduates to be active and involved in health policy....The call now is to...deliver nursing education that ensures all nurses are not only excellent clinicians but are equipped to effectively engage in health policy development and advocacy." Rasheed and colleagues[11(p454)] observed that "Education institutions...should adequately prepare nurses for policy making and nurses should participate in policy making at the organization, system, and national levels." Nursing today exists in a political environment. That is, the profession is influenced directly by governmental rules and laws that affect education, practice, and research. Professional organizations such as the American Nurses Association (ANA) and specialty organizations frequently ask members to write in support of or opposition to proposed legislation that will affect nurses. The need to be knowledgeable about health policy is clear; how can nurse education programs respond? As recently as 2017, Ellenbecker and colleagues[12] developed a staged approach to educating nurses on health policy. They developed comprehensive goals, objectives, a content outline, and student activities for policy courses at the undergraduate and graduate (master's and doctoral) levels. The Toolkit of Policy Resources that accompanies this article offers additional learning activities to engage students in linking policy and practice.

Toolkit of policy resources

This toolkit is a collection of ideas, opportunities, and materials to help nurses move from a novice level of knowledge to more sophisticated, active involvement in nursing policy.

1. *Invest in a textbook.* Textbooks are available in a variety of formats from traditional hardback to interactive digital resources that focus on the process of

---

Box 2
Possible solutions to curricular practice-policy gaps

- Ensure criteria for faculty selection include examples of being politically astute or having a working knowledge of policy, such as faculty who are involved in local and national organizations or serve on committees within those organizations.

- Insist that learning objectives, assessments, learner activities, and competencies are geared toward health policy in course syllabi.

- Enlist faculty from educational departments such as public health, political science, or business faculty to coteach policy.

- Invite policy makers as guest lecturers for policy and clinical courses.

- Orient faculty to updated policy information and provide a toolkit of policy resources for faculty and students.

- Create opportunities within all courses to debate policy issues, analyze current policies, and link policy to practice.

governmental decision-making or provide examples of specific laws, rules, or programs students can analyze. Some textbooks cover the entire policy process from getting problems to government to designing, implementing, and evaluating the response. Some textbooks form an outline for a policy course, complete with political and nurse theory, student activities such as discussion points and case studies, and suggested opportunities for nurse involvement from the level of novice to expert. References are kept up to date in electronic copies of textbooks and point to related resources and websites that may extend one's thinking or perspective about a policy issue.

2. *Join a professional nurse organization.* Many nursing associations and organizations have a policy committee and employ lobbyists to work with members in taking their concerns to policy makers. Membership is voluntary, and involvement depends on one's level of commitment. Nurses should not hesitate to seek participation because they do not have a background in the focus of a committee. This is where many nurses learn about issues, stakeholder roles, support and opposition, and how to function in a policy-making environment. A nurse can build a reputation and improve standing in any committee by attending all sessions, staying alert to news and media on relevant issues, bringing questions to meetings, and generally making oneself a valuable asset to the group.

3. *Join a specialty organization.* Most nurse specialty organizations have legislation or policy committees in which members are encouraged to participate. These groups usually focus on issues that are specific to the group goals (eg, oncology, pediatrics, psychiatric-mental health). Members research pertinent problems and approach policy makers with written position statements. Some groups hire lobbyists, whereas other groups tap members to lobby for concerns. Although in-person meetings were preferred in the past, pandemic-related events caused web-based meetings to become more feasible and widely accepted, extending active involvement in many types of organizations to a greater number of individuals.

4. *Visit a government website.* Government websites are good sources of information. Federal agencies, such as the Department of Health and Human Services (www.hhs.gov),[13] offer a large number and variety of links to health-related sites. A few sites that are pertinent to nurses include www.cdc.gov (Centers for Disease Control),[14] http://www.federalregister.gov/ (Federal Register),[6] and www.nih.gov (National Institutes of Health).[15]

5. *Attend a government hearing.* Some states provide websites where hearings can be attended through a website in real time. For example, Ohio offers Ohiochannel.org where live feeds can be viewed by anyone on the Internet during a governor's address, an agency press conference, or a legislative committee hearing. Remote, digital access to current political processes allows students and faculty to see and hear witnesses who are testifying (and thus discern arguments for support or opposition) and observe the behavior of policy makers during the session. Students are often surprised by what seems to be a lot of movement and talk among policy makers while testimony is being presented.

6. *Register for CE.* CE or Continuing Professional Development programs are available electronically and in person to provide information about targeted issues. These programs also are opportunities where a nurse, as an expert (or even a novice) about an issue, can present information and enlist interest and support. Most programs incorporate a question/answer segment and offer contact hours toward relicensure requirements.

7. *Enroll in a policy course.* Policy courses or presentations may be available at a local university, college, or school. Check the credentials and experience of the presenters and the topics and content for expertise and legitimacy. Moreover, determine if the speaker is presenting an overview of an issue or expects an in-depth dialog with attendees.

8. *Read a variety of journals.* Nursing and other health-related journals often carry recent research or highlight a health problem that needs government attention. Although not all problems are within the government's purview, sometimes a solution to one problem will stimulate its application to a related problem. For example, an article may focus on access to care related to transportation, yet access to care may also be related to Internet bandwidth in remote areas. Special editions of journals may highlight the level of interest in a subject and may identify researchers or others who share similar interests.

9. *Join nonhealth-related interest groups.* Nonhealth-related organizations, such as the League of Women Voters, present symposia or seminars on specific topics through webinars and podcasts. These are usually nonbiased, balanced presentations in which at least 2 perspectives are presented.

10. *Check for bias.* Some organizations offer sessions that are overtly or covertly biased on an issue related to health policy. It can be instructive to attend both biased and unbiased sessions to ascertain what the arguments are in support or opposition to an issue. It is important to assess the rationale of opponents to an issue of interest to understand and counter their arguments.

11. *Attend a local government meeting.* Government entities, such as city councils or county commissioners, may provide open meetings to obtain a sense of the importance of an issue to constituents. Citizens are encouraged to share their views and suggestions by testifying at the meetings.

12. *Write a letter to the editor.* Students and practicing nurses can write letters to an editor for a variety of venues including local newspapers or scholarly journals. Keep letters to one page and address only one issue. Identify yourself as a nurse and sign the letter with your name and credentials.

13. *Write an op ed.* Newspaper op ed (opposite the editorial page) sections, not affiliated with the editorial board, encourage thoughtful considerations or perspectives on an issue or problem. These narrative features that express an author's position invite response and can stimulate discussion among colleagues and, as a result of replies to the authors, can expand your interest group.

14. *Contact your policy maker.* Many textbooks, hardcover or electronic, offer chapters with specific directions to get in touch with local, state, and federal policy makers and engage in policy activities. The US government also provides contact information for federal, state, and local elected officials online (www.usa.gov/elected-officials).

15. *Prepare an elevator speech.* An elevator speech is a 60-second oral presentation that identifies who you are, what your issue or problem is, why it is important, and what you want from the policy maker. An elevator speech allows you to capture the interest of a policy maker quickly, make your point, and pique the listener's interest, so a more in-depth discussion can follow at a later time. Nurses should practice their elevator speeches so they can be recalled quickly when the opportunity arises.

16. *Use talking points.* Talking points, a 1-page document that summarizes an issue, can be given to a policy maker after a personal or phone visit. Keep words short and nonmedical, use no more than 2 different fonts, be judicious with color (black type on white paper is easy to read), and do not use scented paper or paper with distractions, such as designs with flowers or animals.

17. *Maintain professional social media profiles.* Keep all profiles up to date in LinkedIn, Twitter, and other professional organizational sites. It is important to establish a professional persona across all social media to build the reputation necessary to influence policy.

Leadership Role of the Basic and Advanced Nurse

The role of the basic and advanced nurse in health policy begins with knowledge of the policy process at the local, state, or federal levels. Degrees of involvement are much like Benner's model[16] in which a practitioner can increase skill and sophistication. The first step is to develop awareness of policy as a part of every aspect of nursing, and then the nurse can choose the area, topic, and depth of personal involvement. It is especially important for novices to engage with other nurses who have an interest in policy. Develop a network of colleagues, professional organizations, and specialty organizations. A baccalaureate student may begin to identify a clinical problem that government could help solve. Master's and doctoral students can become actively involved in policy by presenting testimony at a hearing or attending an Interested Parties meeting with a proposal for solutions. The advanced nurse can focus on a clinical issue in a professional project, thesis, or doctoral dissertation. A DNP-prepared nurse can identify clinical problems and collaborate with a PhD-prepared researcher to conduct a study that addresses an important problem. Nurses who are involved in policy making are typically involved in the implementation phase rather than agenda setting, design, or evaluation.[11] By limiting their involvement to the policy implementation phase, nurses miss opportunities to put issues on government agendas and recommend public programs for evaluation by relevant agencies for effectiveness and efficiency.

Emerging Issues

Below are issues nurses need to consider when they want to get more involved in policy making.

1. *Rapid growth of telehealth.* Fink[17] asserts that telehealth is the number-one change in the future of health care resulting from the COVID-19 pandemic. Health-care providers such as Advanced Practice Registered Nurses (APRNs), physicians, and physician's associates are screening, triaging, diagnosing, treating, monitoring, and evaluating patients through remote technology. Telehealth is bringing health care to those who may not have had access due to gaps in social determinants of health and other factors. An example of a nurse at the forefront of the intersection of technology, practice, and education is Debi Samsel, DNP. She and a team of 3 other faculty members (medical engineer, nutritionist, and health informaticist) at the University of Cincinnati (OH) have invented a drone that holds a camera with screen and a cargo box that delivers medical supplies and self-administered tests directly to patient homes. Dr Samsel tested the drone in a senior living apartment. The drone was developed to assist in managing chronic diseases, postoperative care, health coaching, and consultation.[18] This example clearly illustrates why health policies need to stay up to date to match current health-care practice.
2. *Renewed attention to health policy.* The COVID-19 pandemic revealed a lack of understanding on the part of the general population about the policy process.[19] Some citizens were confused when policies changed as science evolved.[19] Scientists and organizations were accused of lacking credibility when announcing data and trends, and misinformation and disinformation about so-called treatments and cures filled social media.[19] Scrutinizing policies governing the process of

identifying, tracing, developing, testing, disseminating, monitoring, and evaluating the virus exposed a lack of knowledge about how policy decisions are made and highlighted a need for more education.

3. *Explosion of technology.* Some who distrusted policy directives and vaccines because of the rapidity of their development may not have fully grasped the magnitude by which science has expanded during the years. When measles and polio were studied, laboratories often consisted of a Bunsen burner, agar plate, and test tubes. Currently, laboratories are equipped with technologically advanced equipment, highly educated scientists, and enormous public and private sector funding. Researchers followed standard testing (laboratory, animal, clinical) protocols.[20] Researchers also had the ability to collect large data sets because of the technology available today. Policy decisions, in part, were based on current ability to rely on big data.

4. *Rethinking assessment approaches in nurse education.* Nurse educators are challenged with providing learning opportunities relevant to current world events. Many nursing programs were already well-positioned to offer online education when the pandemic began. A move toward competency-based education is overcoming time and geographic boundaries that limited traditional nursing education. Competency-based education will produce a new generation of nurses who have been educated differently. Rather than expecting a student to master a concept or skill in an academic term, competence will be measured throughout an academic program at progressively increasing levels of complexity.[9]

5. *New models for nurse education.* Educators are cognizant of the need for a more diverse workforce and a greater emphasis on assuring equitable provision of health care to diverse populations. Evidence-informed and evidence-based practice is replacing "that's-the-way-we've-always-done-it" approach to providing nursing care.[21] Nurses are taught to think critically, analyze deeply, identify human patterns of behavior, maintain ethical standards, and practice within a holistic, caring framework. Baccalaureate education is becoming the entry level for professional nursing in lieu of hospital diploma or associate degree. Policy and technology have tremendous potential to support modern approaches to nurse education that prepare future nurses for success in an increasingly challenging and dynamic health-care environment.

6. *E practice roles.* Nurses have carved out practices in arenas that were not considered the domain of nurses even a few years ago. Nurses are innovators and inventors, policy analysts, university presidents, board chairs, experts in direct care, and leaders in health-care systems. APRNs today are limited to 4 areas of practice: clinical nurse specialist, nurse practitioner, nurse midwife, and nurse anesthetist. However, based on the current state and projected trajectory of technology and practice, those roles are likely to continue to expand in scope and expertise. The challenge is in helping individual nurses incorporate policy, education, and technology into their own unique practice environment.

SUMMARY

This article links nurse practice with public and private sector policy decisions as an integral component of professional leadership. The authors contend that nursing exists in a political environment. That is, governmental laws and regulations and private sector policies have a direct impact on nurse practice. The educational curriculum must prepare students to identify health-policy issues and health-systems problems. A toolkit of resources is presented to assist students and practicing nurses to work with policy makers in designing, implementing, and evaluating policies and programs. Classroom simulation, drones, and other computerized devices highlight the importance of the effective use of technology for current and future practice. The intersection of education, technology, policy, and practice positions the nurse to exert influence on officials in the government and the boardroom. Engagement in policy making is critical to completely fulfilling the role of the professional nurse.

CLINICS CARE POINTS

- Nurses need to recognize the reciprocal impact of technology and practice and be prepared to support quality of care by influencing policy decisions.

- Without a strong focus on the process of policy making in the nurse education curricula, nurses will not be prepared to make sustainable change for the profession or be effective leaders in the boardroom.

- Integration of competencies in linking policy to practice throughout curricula at all levels of nursing education is essential to the development of effective nurse leaders.

- Practical tools and strategies to support nurse involvement in policy making include membership in nursing organizations, attendance at virtual policy meetings, contact with government policy makers, and submissions to scholarly publications and media.

- Emerging issues in nurse education and technology present rich opportunities to become more involved in the policy-making process and influence the future of nursing.

DISCLOSURE

The authors whose names are listed above certify that they have NO affiliations with or involvement in any organization or entity with any financial interest (such as honoraria; educational grants; participation in speakers' bureaus; membership, employment, consultancies, stock ownership, or other equity interest; and expert testimony or patent-licensing arrangements) or nonfinancial interest (such as personal or professional relationships, affiliations, knowledge, or beliefs) in the subject matter or materials discussed in this article.

REFERENCES

1. Nightingale F. Notes on nursing: what it is, and what it is not. Independently Published 2020;1820–910.
2. Importance of policies and procedures for hospitals. PowerDMS website 2020. Available at: https://www.powerdms.com/policy-learning-center/importance-of-policies-and-procedures-for-hospitals. Accessed September 26, 2021.
3. About the NLC. National Council of State Boards of Nursing website. 2021. Available at: https://ncsbn.org/16277.html. Accessed on December 7, 2021.
4. Transportation and health tool. U.S. Department of Transportation. 2021. Available at: https://www.transportation.gov/transportation-health-tool. Accessed on December 13, 2021.
5. Strategies for changing policies. Institute for patient and family centered care website. 2020. Available at: https://www.ipfcc.org/bestpractices/Strategies-for-Changing-Policies.pdf. Accessed October 28, 2021.
6. Daily Journal of the United States Government. Federal Register website 2021. Available at: https://www.federalregister.gov/. Accessed December 7, 2021.
7. Indicators. Centers for Disease Control and Prevention website. 2021. Available at: https://www.cdc.gov/eval/indicators/index.htm. Accessed December 2, 2021.

8. Rural Health Policy.. Rural Health Information Hub website. 2021. Available at: https://www.ruralhealthinfo.org/topics/rural-health-policy#policymaking-process. Accessed on October 16, 2021.

9. The essentials: Core competencies for professional nursing education. Am Assoc Colleges Nurs website 2021. Available at: https://www.aacnnursing.org/Portals/42/AcademicNursing/pdf/Essentials-2021.pdf. Accessed on October 13, 2021.

10. De Cordova PB, Steck MBW, Vermeesch A, et al. Health policy engagement among graduate nursing students in the United States. Nurs Forum 2019;54: 38–44.

11. Rasheed DP, Younas A, Mehdi F. Challenges, extent of involvement, and the impact of nurses' involvement in politics and policy making in the last two decades: an integrative review, 2020 integrative review. J Nurs Scholarsh 2020; 54(4):446–55.

12. Ellenbecker CH, Fawcett J, Jones EJ, et al. A staged approach to educating nurses in health policy, staged approach to educating nurses in health policy. Policy, Politics, & Nursing Practice, 2017. Practice 2017;18(1):44–56.

13. U.S. Department of Health and Human Services. U.S. Department of Health and Human Services website. 2021. Available at: www.hhs.gov. Accessed on December 13, 2021.

14. Centers for Disease Control and Prevention. Centers for disease control and prevention website 2021. Available at: www.cdc.gov. Accessed on January 6, 2022.

15. National Institutes of Health. National Institutes of Health website 2021. Available at: www.nih.gov. Accessed on January 6, 2022.

16. Petiprin A. Biography and career of Dr. Patricia Benner. Nursing Theory website 2020. Available at: https://nursing-theory.org/nursing-theorists/Patricia-Benner.php. Accessed on February 3, 2022.

17. Fink JLW. 8 Ways COVID-19 will change the future of healthcare. Health Grades website 2021. Available at: https://www.healthgrades.com/pro/8-ways-covid-19-will-change-the-future-of-healthcare. Accessed on September 26, 2021.

18. New UC telehealth drone makes house calls. University of Cincinnati website 2021. Available at: https://www.uc.edu/news/articles/2021/03/virtual-medicine-new-uc-telehealth-drone-makes-house-calls.html. Accessed on September 26, 2021.

19. How to address COVID-19 vaccine misinformation. Centers Dis Control Prev website 2021. Available at: https://www.cdc.gov/vaccines/covid-19/health-departments/addressing-vaccine-misinformation.html. Accessed January 6, 2022.

20. Developing COVID-19 vaccines. Centers Dis Control Prev website 2021. Available at: https://www.cdc.gov/coronavirus/2019-ncov/vaccines/distributing/steps-ensure-safety.html. Accessed December 2, 2021.

21. Theofanidis D. Evidence based nursing: barriers and challenges for contemporary nurses, 2021 nurses. Health Res J 2021;7(1):1–3. Available at: https://ejournals.epublishing.ekt.gr/index.php/HealthResJ/article/viewFile/26093/21262. Accessed on September 26, 2021.

Interprofessional Simulation in a Digital World

Teaching Collaborative Practice in Web-Based Environments

Lisa Rohrig, MS, RN, CHSE, CHSOS[a],*, Stephanie Burlingame, RN, BSN[b],
Miranda Bertie Dickerson, MS, RN, CHSE[c],
Edith A. Harter, BSN, RN, CHSE[b], Stephanie Justice, DNP, RN, CHSE[d]

KEYWORDS

- Educational technology • Feedback • Interdisciplinary communication
- Interprofessional education • Nursing education • Patient care team
- Patient simulation • Simulation training

KEY POINTS

- Interprofessional competencies are important to all nursing and health science curricula and are mandated by some of the bodies that regulate health care programs.
- Simulation is an effective teaching strategy to prepare students for interprofessional practice.
- Interprofessional simulations can be conducted successfully through web-based teleconferencing platforms.
- Transitioning in-person interprofessional simulations to teleconferencing formats requires careful planning.

[a] Technology Learning Complex, Ohio State University College of Nursing Columbus, Room 298 Newton Hall, 1585 Neil Avenue, Columbus, OH 43210, USA; [b] Skills and Simulation Faculty, Technology Learning Complex, Ohio State University College of Nursing Columbus, Room 288 Newton Hall, 1585 Neil Avenue, Columbus, OH 43210, USA; [c] Technology Learning Complex, Ohio State University College of Nursing Columbus, Room 288 Newton Hall, 1585 Neil Avenue, Columbus, OH 43210, USA; [d] Ohio State University College of Nursing Columbus, Room 288 Newton Hall, 1585 Neil Avenue, Columbus, OH 43210, USA
* Corresponding author.
E-mail address: Rohrig.1@osu.edu

Nurs Clin N Am 57 (2022) 639–652
https://doi.org/10.1016/j.cnur.2022.06.011
0029-6465/22/Published by Elsevier Inc.

nursing.theclinics.com

BACKGROUND

In 2010, the World Health Organization (WHO) called for interprofessional collaboration in health care education as a necessary step to prepare a practice-ready health care workforce ready to deliver the highest level of care.[1] The Interprofessional Education Collaborative (IPEC), which represents 21 national health professions associations,[2] has outlined core competencies for interprofessional education (IPE) for health science students.[3] In a systematic review, Aldriwest and colleagues[4] found that simulation-based learning, e-learning, and problem-based learning were the most common approaches to IPE. Further, IPE results in enhanced teamwork, collaboration, and an understanding of individual health care roles within patient care.[5]

The American Association of Colleges of Nursing 2021 Essentials (core curricular elements) for entry-level professional nursing education contains two competency domains that are directly related to IPE. These are Domain 6: Interprofessional Partnerships and Domain 8: Informatics and Healthcare Technologies.[6] Domain 6 describes interprofessional partnerships as intentional collaboration with health care team members and other stakeholders to improve health care outcomes.[6] Domain 8 describes learning opportunities that integrate informatics and communication technologies into the provision of care and decision-making to improve safety, quality, and efficiency according to best practices and standards.[6] Students participating in IPE simulations have opportunities to participate in collaborative learning that fulfills both domains through well-developed, focused, and faculty-facilitated IPE simulations.

IPE can be difficult to carry out in a university setting due to varying class and clinical schedules for each profession. Yune and colleagues[7] investigated IPE with faculty from medicine, nursing, and pharmacy and discovered that 95.8% of faculty had no experience with IPE, despite believing that it was necessary. Knowing the value of IPE is not enough to overcome the barriers to implementing IPE. The logistics of scheduling multiple groups of students from different health professions for an in-person IPE experience in one physical location is challenging. Now more than ever, with ongoing threats of significant interruption to in-person learning by a widespread pandemic event or other disaster, health education faculty need to be prepared to deliver IPE in a variety of flexible formats that accommodate the largest number of learners possible. Faculty and staff commitment to planning and developing IPE learning activities is essential to the success of web-based IPE simulation experiences.[8] In this article, we present a case study of how an established in-person IPE simulation program was transitioned to a web-based videoconference environment in response to the coronavirus disease (COVID-19). Recommendations for preparation, orientation, setup, roles, simulation workflow, debriefing, and evaluation are provided for health care educators who are considering flexible IPE simulation formats.

THE EXCELLENCE IN INTERPROFESSIONAL SIMULATION EDUCATION: A CASE STUDY
History of the Excellence in Interprofessional Simulation Education

The Excellence in Interprofessional Simulation Education (ECLIPSE) program was established through a grassroots effort at the university. Faculty representatives from six health science programs (nursing, pharmacy, advanced practice nursing, physical therapy, respiratory therapy, and medical dietetics) came together to plan an in-person IPE simulation for their students in the spring of 2012. The inaugural simulations involved a total of 150 students who were evenly distributed by profession into 20 groups. The planning committee developed two complex acute care patient care scenarios that would be realistic, offer meaningful clinical experience to students, and foster collaboration between students from different professions. Each professional program involved in the simulation had a faculty representative who contributed to the development of the simulation scenarios. Representation by every participating health care profession in scenario development was essential to ensure the role of the profession and scope of practice were accurately represented in the scenarios. The simulation format, schedule, and selection of target student populations within each academic program, student orientation, and simulation evaluation measures were developed during those six months of planning by the team. The ECLIPSE learning objectives reflected the IPEC core competencies and included:

1. Create a climate of mutual respect and understanding
2. Understand the roles and responsibilities of other professions
3. Develop interprofessional communication skills
4. Develop an interprofessional plan of care

The Excellence in Interprofessional Simulation Education In-Person Simulation

ECLIPSE has expanded in the past 10 years and currently reaches over 400 students representing 12 health and social science programs each semester. Programs include undergraduate nursing; advanced practice clinical nurse leader and acute care nurse practitioner; medicine; physical therapy; occupational therapy; respiratory therapy and advanced practice respiratory therapy; medical dietetics; social work; pharmacy; and speech pathology. Four patient scenarios have now been developed for use with the ECLIPSE simulation program. Existing cases include patients with challenging health and social situations, such as multiple comorbidities, low health literacy, mental health conditions, and compounding social determinants of health.

The simulation is conducted in person in the College of Nursing's Technology Learning Complex (TLC), a nursing clinical simulation and skills center staffed by five nurses with TLC faculty roles. Student groups participate in a 3-hour multidisciplinary simulation experience in a TLC simulation laboratory. Volunteer faculty from each health care profession facilitate the simulations by offering support to students without interfering with their experiential learning. Their goal in facilitation is to ensure learning objectives are met and allow students time to think critically and independently by providing guidance only when needed. In addition to faculty facilitators from each profession, the IPE simulation relies on the TLC simulation faculty to manage the medical moulage, environment set up, and operation of simulation technology.

The TLC faculties are responsible for all standardized patient (SP) actors utilized in simulation as well. An ECLIPSE committee member is assigned as the simulation room moderator to ensure adherence to the simulation schedule, evaluate the team's performance, and lead the debriefing discussion at the end of simulations. Students are provided with an extended orientation to the event within their online modules the week before simulations. All students, faculty, and actors involved in ECLIPSE receive onsite orientation as well. Students complete team and simulation evaluation tools. Room moderators receive a debriefing tool and complete a faculty version of the team evaluation tool.

COVID-19 was declared a pandemic on March 10, 2020, by the WHO.[9] Masks, social distancing, and stay-at-home orders have become commonplace throughout the world. The Centers for Disease Control recommended keeping six feet of space between individuals when it was not possible to stay home. Before the pandemic, ECLIPSE simulations were conducted in a simulation laboratory with two SPs and up to 30 people in a simulation room. Social distancing protocols were not possible with that number of people in the available space. Moreover, the pandemic caused all didactic courses to shift to an online-only format, and no in-person simulations or laboratories were permitted at the university after the pandemic began. Academic administrators were on the verge of making the difficult decision to cancel the ECLIPSE program for the rest of the academic year.

To avoid canceling IPE simulations entirely, ECLIPSE faculty strategized to convert an in-person acute care setting, multipatient, multidisciplinary simulation to a videoconferencing platform. Converting classes to online formats, including IPE classes, is not unique to Ohio State. For example, an in-person IPE course was converted to an online format using online synchronous meetings and discussion boards for student reflection at Oregon Health & Science University.[10] However, the ECLIPSE faculty aimed to preserve the simulation component in IPE experiences because they felt that simulation, even if it was less realistic than the in-person experience, was essential to provide students with an authentic learning context in which achievement of learning objectives could be clearly demonstrated.

Transition to Web-Based Format

Transitioning from an in-person simulation to a virtual environment is an arduous task. Considering the large number of stakeholders from 12 different health professions, varying levels of personal familiarity with technology, and the complex interactions that occur in in-person simulations can make the task seem overwhelming. We chose Zoom as our videoconferencing platform for the ECLIPSE simulation because the university had already provided accounts for all students and employees, and Zoom had already been proven to be reliable with ample support. However, the TLC simulation faculty had little experience with Zoom before its implementation with ECLIPSE. Becoming experts on Zoom videoconference technology was imperative to conducting a successful virtual simulation of this magnitude.

In the four months before launching web-based ECLIPSE simulations, TLC faculty conducted several informal practice sessions. TLC faculty logged in from different devices and practiced sharing the orientation video and simulation documents and assigning breakout rooms in Zoom. They determined that students needed to utilize a fully charged laptop or desktop computer rather than a tablet or smart phone because Zoom features are not fully functional on mobile devices and are less functional with Zoom. For optimal simulation flow and adequate direction and assistance for SPs, TLC faculty planned to set up the simulation with the faculty moderator and co-moderator and the SP actor socially distanced in the simulation laboratory. Moulage was applied quickly by TLC faculty while both the faculty and SP were masked, and the SP did some of their own preparation for the simulation as well. Ventilators and other medical equipment were situated in the laboratory scenario as they would have been for an in-person simulation. Laptop and iPad cameras were set up to broadcast the scene to Zoom participants. TLC and disciplinary faculty planned to moderate the online simulations and intermittently communicate with patient actors who were positioned in hospital beds on opposite sides of large simulation rooms. Further adjustments were made to prevent feedback echoes through moderator laptops while SPs spoke to students in simulation on laptops at the bedside (**Fig. 1**).

The TLC faculty tested their setup to determine how realistically they had recreated aspects of the in-person simulation. The extensive testing sessions gave TLC faculty a better understanding of Zoom host abilities, recording options, and the expected student experience in the format. TLC faculty spent a substantial amount of time trying different Zoom views and settings to determine which ones allowed students to see the SP and as many of their peer participants as possible. It was through this trial-

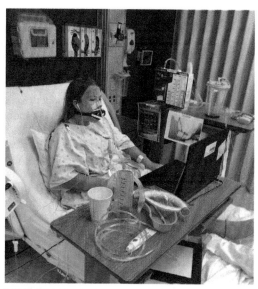

Fig. 1. Standardized Patient.

and-error process that TLC faculty identified important settings and features in Zoom that needed to be used in videoconference simulations, such as assigning breakout rooms by profession and having a moderator answer questions in the text chat so the flow of the simulation was not disrupted (**Fig. 2**).

Specific roles and responsibilities of moderator and co-moderator and SP actors were established, such as who would admit students to the Zoom meeting room, take attendance, maintain the schedule, share documents, and answer chat questions. The necessary equipment and optimal setup of the mock patient room were decided. Once TLC faculty felt competent in the structure and flow of ECLIPSE simulations in Zoom, several dress-rehearsal sessions were scheduled 2 weeks before the first simulation for all profession faculty facilitators. During these dress rehearsals, TLC faculty performed all operations related to the upcoming simulations, such as opening a Zoom meeting, assigning faculty facilitators to breakout rooms, sharing

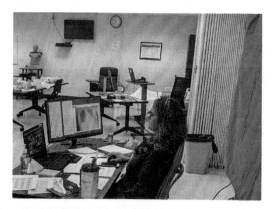

Fig. 2. Facilitator.

the orientation video, and describing the proposed timeline of events. Facilitators asked questions about Zoom capabilities and made suggestions regarding patient moulage. All aspects of the simulation and timeline were finalized during these faculty facilitator orientation sessions.

The 30-minute in-person orientation for student participants, which had traditionally been delivered as a PowerPoint presentation in the in-person ECLIPSE simulations, was replaced with a prerecorded orientation presentation for the web-based simulations. The presentation introduced students to the Zoom videoconference interface and explained to students how to interact with the SP and peers from other professions in Zoom, including how to raise their Zoom "hands" if they had a question or comment. The orientation presentation also covered the simulation timeline and how to enter and leave the Zoom breakout rooms. Students were instructed to rename themselves in the Zoom participant list using the following format: "Profession-Name," for example, "RT-Betsy." Faculties renamed themselves in Zoom as "Faculty-Profession-Name," for example, "Faculty-Pharmacy-Dr. Smith." This naming convention provided organization and transparency related to professional identities and roles during simulations.

The same patient story and documentation were used for the web-based simulation as the one that had been used for the in-person simulation. The SP actor logged into the Zoom room on a laptop placed on the bedside table or on their lap while in the patient bed. They renamed themselves in Zoom as "Patient-Name," for example, "Patient-Ann Arbor." The patient's video was also "spotlighted" in Zoom so that she was always in view during the simulation. The simulated patient rooms mimicked the in-person scenarios but had adjustments that allowed easy viewing of various aspects of the patient and their environment through video streaming. For example, a ventilator was positioned at the SP's bedside, and the ventilator circuit tubing was hidden behind the patient's bed. Screenshots of ventilator displays were used during the simulation when students needed that information.

Videoconferencing equipment, such as iPads, laptops, headphones, and rolling iPad tripod holders, were tested during practice sessions to determine which combination would best allow the SP to display their wound dressings, medical equipment, monitor, and inserted lines and drains without assistance from the moderator (to maintain social distance). When students from any profession wanted to assess, talk to, or implement care for the patient, they raised their virtual Zoom hands. The moderator called on the students in the order they raised their hands. If the student wanted to see a certain part of the patient or scene, for example, the chest tube or an incision, the SP actor pointed her iPad camera at the item or showed a picture of the item.

TLC faculty also used creative strategies to simulate patient medical records. In the in-person simulation, all students from participating professions reviewed paper-based patient charts in binders on tables in their simulation rooms. In the web-based simulation format, portable document format versions of the medical records were provided in online modules students completed before simulation and shared as links in the chat box during simulation for student reference. Laboratory and radiology results were also provided in the chat by the co-moderator.

Orientation and Preparation

Student orientation

Students are required to complete a five-module, asynchronous, online course delivered through the university's learning management system (Canvas course) before they attend any ECLIPSE interprofessional simulation, regardless of whether it is delivered in an in-person or web-based format. Participating students from each health care profession choose a simulation session that fits their schedule through an online event organization and signup tool to ensure equal representation of all participating professions within each ECLIPSE simulation session. Students are placed in a Canvas course corresponding to their chosen session. This allows them the opportunity to meet and interact virtually with other team members who will attend their session and discuss topics related to the simulation objectives.

The online presimulation course introduces concepts from the Team Strategies and Tools to Enhance Performance and Patient Safety (Team STEPPS), an evidence-based IPE and training program. Key Team STEPPS principles include communication, leadership, situational monitoring, mutual support, and shared decision-making.[11,12] Other important resources are also provided for the students through the course, including an orientation video; a video example of bedside rounding; the introduction, situation, background, assessment, recommendations communication tool; simulated patient medical records; and a post-simulation reflection/evaluation.

Faculty orientation

All faculties received orientation to the simulations by viewing a recorded orientation video before participation. The faculty orientation overviews the program's background, objectives, and schedule. It also reviews simulation facilitation best practices. Simulation involves experiential learning; so, faculty must learn to operate as facilitators of student-led learning in the safe environment that simulation is designed to provide. Faculties are discouraged from "relecturing" or telling students what to do in simulation; rather, they are encouraged to use open-ended questions to allow students to make independent decisions. With the regular additions of new faculty in ECLIPSE, requiring completion of a faculty orientation ensures a more uniform experience for all students.

Standardized patient actor orientation

The TLC faculties maintain a database of SP actors for simulations. Many SPs are community members, university students, or personally known by simulation faculty. Social media and word of mouth have helped establish this list of individuals over several years. Individuals who fit the simulated patient demographics were contacted to determine interest and availability to participate in the simulations. Information about the patient's background, history, and hospital stay, as well as responses to expected student questions, were provided to the SPs. TLC faculties recorded an introduction video showing what equipment would be used, how moulage would be applied, and an orientation to the room and equipment. Additionally, the SPs were provided with information about the videoconferencing program that would be used and offered a chance to familiarize themselves with the activity and expectations just before the simulation. They were shown how to use the iPad camera to allow the students to view equipment, monitors, or themselves when prompted. Ample time was provided before the beginning of each simulation to practice with the equipment and technology and answer any questions.

The patient was trained to provide assessment findings in several ways. The students talked directly with the patient and verbalized interventions and assessments step-by-step so that students in other professions could learn what they do. If the student wanted an assessment finding, such as lung sounds, they asked the patient, who verbally reported them on cue. Assessment results would be verbalized by the moderator when the patient was in the "intubated" state. Patient actors also provided feedback about team performance from a patient's perspective in debriefing. Following simulations, SPs were paid via an electronic gift card.

Web-Based Simulation Workflow

After 3 to 4 months of careful planning and testing, the web-based ECLISPE simulation was ready for its first run. The main Zoom room simulated all the students, faculty, and SPs being together in real life. The moderator, co-moderator, and patient—who were physically in the same simulation laboratory space—also stayed in the main Zoom room throughout the simulation. Zoom breakout rooms were labeled by profession (eg, nursing, pharmacy, or social work) to designate which students would be assigned to each room by the moderator.

During in-person simulations, if students had questions for a student from another profession, they would simply walk through the physical space and talk to them. To prevent confusion in communications in the web-based videoconference environment, breakout rooms served as the space for students in each profession to "huddle" among themselves, review the medical record, and discuss their profession-specific care plans. If students from one profession had a question for those from a different profession, they were instructed to enter the main Zoom room, raise their Zoom hand, and wait for the moderator to call on them. They also had the option to ask their questions in the chat box in the main room. The student from the other profession would simply respond to the question if they were in the main Zoom room, or if they were in a profession-specific breakout room, the moderator summoned them to come to the main Zoom room to collaborate with their peer who had the question.

The simulation faculties designed the web-based simulation to follow the same schedule as the one set for the original in-person simulations. The schedule was as follows:

1. Orientation (30 minutes)
2. Professional huddles (within professions) to discuss patient history and plan of care (10 minutes)
3. Collaborative bedside rounding on patient, including students from all disciplines (40 minutes)
4. Implementation of the treatment plan by individual professions and collaboration among professions as necessary (40 minutes)
5. Combined rerounding, including all professions (30 minutes)
6. Debriefing the simulation and completion of evaluations (30 minutes)

A medical student or nurse practitioner student from one profession led rounds as they did in the in-person simulations and called out one student from each profession in turn to give their patient report and recommendations for care. During or immediately following rounds, new orders were written in the chat by students for all to reference for implementation. Following the first collaborative bedside round, students took turns talking with the patient and implementing care as described earlier by raising their Zoom hands. During this phase of the simulation, different professions were going in and out of their disciplinary breakout rooms, while some stayed in the main room and observed other professions interacting with the patient. At a predetermined time, students convened as a team in the main Zoom room for a second combined rounding session on the patient.

Debriefing followed the second collaborative rounding session and was facilitated by the room moderator, utilizing the same questions as the in-person simulations. Debriefing sessions were conducted with the whole group in one room. Moderators would ensure that all student and professional voices were heard. Faculty from each profession and the patient actor provided feedback to the students about the team's performance. Links to simulation evaluation surveys, including a team evaluation and a separate simulation evaluation, were posted in the Zoom text chat and completed by students during the debriefing phase.

Program Evaluation

The TLC has utilized the modified Simulation Effectiveness Tool (SET-M) to evaluate simulations since its inception. The SET-M is a validated 19-item tool with a 3-point Likert scale (1 = "Do not agree," 3 = "Strongly agree"), which measures student-reported effectiveness of simulations within the subcategories of prebriefing, scenario, and debriefing.[13] During all previous academic years, when ECLIPSE simulations were conducted in person, the SET-M results were overwhelmingly positive. The web-based simulations were also rated highly by students, although the ratings were overall slightly lower (**Table 1**).

When comparing the SET-M results between the two simulation formats (virtual and in-person), a slight decrease in average ratings was observed for most of the items (see **Table 1**). However, the two prebriefing SET-M items were rated higher for virtual simulations than in person. The overall mean SET-M score for web-based simulations was 2.71, a decrease from in-person simulations of 0.04. Comments on the web-based SET-M evaluations were also overwhelmingly positive, with two main themes indicating students found value in learning from and collaborating with the health care team.

A modified version of the Performance Assessment of Communication and Teamwork (PACT) tool, which was developed within the Team STEPPS program, has also been used to evaluate ECLIPSE simulations. The novice version of the PACT was administered to students participating in both in-person and web-based simulations to allow them to evaluate their team's performance. The PACT is divided into five sections, including team structure, leadership, situational monitoring, mutual support, and communication. Students used the PACT tool to rate how well their team performed in each of the domains and provide optional comments for each domain (**Fig. 3**).

Due to decreased realism in the web-based simulation setting, the ECLIPSE faculties expected these scores to drop, and they did. Students could not put their hands on the patients to perform their assessments and procedures; instead, they described procedures step-by-step for other students. This facilitated some collaborative learning by allowing students to visualize the procedures through the descriptions by their peers. However, it was less than ideal. As with the SET-M outcomes, the average ratings on the PACT were lower for the virtual simulations than the in-person ratings, but they remained relatively high. The overall average means were 4.53 for in-person and 4.35 for web-based ECLISE simulations, demonstrating a 0.18 decrease for virtual (**Table 2**). Both the SET-M and PACT evaluations were administered in electronic format using Qualtrics, and students could complete the evaluations on their computers or smartphones. PACT surveys were completed by students at the beginning of debrief sessions to prompt them to contribute their thoughts about team performance to the discussion. SET-M surveys were provided at the end of debrief sessions as these surveys included questions about the effectiveness of debriefing as part of simulation.

DISCUSSION

When factors, such as scheduling, physical location, and interruptions in normal academic practice jeopardize in-person interprofessional simulation experiences, web-based interprofessional simulations offer opportunities to preserve continuity in IPE

Table 1
Simulation effectiveness tool—modified the Excellence in Interprofessional Simulation Education in-person and virtual sims comparison

	Mean Score In-Person Sims	Mean Score Virtual Sims	Changes
Prebriefing:			
Prebriefing increased my confidence.	2.70	2.82	+0.12
Prebriefing was beneficial to my learning.	2.78	2.84	+0.06
Scenarios			
I am better prepared to respond to changes in my patient's condition.	2.78	2.74	−0.04
I developed a better understanding of the pathophysiology.	2.52	2.51	−0.01
I am more confident of my nursing assessment skills.	2.72	2.60	−0.12
I felt empowered to make clinical decisions.	2.80	2.75	−0.05
I developed a better understanding of medications.	2.45	2.45	Unchanged
I had the opportunity to practice my clinical decision-making skills.	2.89	2.85	−0.04
I am more confident in my ability to prioritize care and interventions.	2.80	2.78	−0.02
I am more confident in communicating with my patient.	2.82	2.66	−0.16
I am more confident in my ability to teach patients about their illness and interventions.	2.72	2.59	−0.13
I am more confident in my ability to report information to health care team.	2.84	2.84	Unchanged
I am more confident in providing interventions that foster patient safety.	2.78	2.72	−0.06
I am more confident in using evidence-based practice to provide care.	2.68	2.66	−0.02
Debriefing			
Debriefing contributed to my learning.	2.82	2.73	−0.09
Debriefing allowed me to verbalize my feelings before focusing on the scenario.	2.77	2.71	−0.06
Debriefing was valuable in helping me improve my clinical judgment.	2.78	2.71	−0.07
Debriefing provided opportunities to self-reflect on my performance during simulation.	2.84	2.80	−0.04
Debriefing was a constructive evaluation of the simulation.	2.83	2.79	−0.04
Overall mean	2.75	2.71	−0.04
Overall median	2.78	2.73	−0.05

3 = Strongly Agree, 2 = Agree, and 1 = Do Not Agree.

while meeting curricular requirements imposed by accreditors and other organizations that regulate academic health care education. The ECLIPSE simulations were originally designed as rounding experiences in an acute-care setting and are more realistic in an in-person simulation compared to a web-based simulation. Though telemedicine

Performance Assessment for Communication and Teamwork (PACT) Simulation Observational Tool
Novice Observer Form

W CENTER FOR HEALTH SCIENCES INTERPROFESSIONAL
EDUCATION. RESEARCH & PRACTICE
UNIVERSITY of WASHINGTON

Profession: Med Nurs Pharm PA other:_____   **Date:**_____

Scenario: 1st 2nd 3rd   **Scenario Type:** SVT CHF Asthma OB Peds _____   **Session:** AM PM

From your perspective as a team observer, how would you describe the perfomance of this team? You are not describing the performance of individuals, except with regard to how they influence team performance. You are instead describing team functioning.

TeamSTEPPS Skill Domains	Poor		Average		Excellent	Comments?
Team Structure	❏	❏	❏	❏	❏	
identifies goals, assigns roles and responsibilities, holds members accountable						
Leadership	❏	❏	❏	❏	❏	
utilizes resources, delegates tasks and balances workload, conducts briefs, huddles, and debriefs, empowers members to speak freely						
Situation Monitoring	❏	❏	❏	❏	❏	
includes patient/family in communication, cross monitors members and applies the STEP process, fosters communication						
Mutual Support	❏	❏	❏	❏	❏	
advocates for the patient, resolves conflict using Two-Challenge rule, CUS and DESC Script, works collaboratively						
Communication	❏	❏	❏	❏	❏	
provides brief, clear, specific and timely information, seeks and communicates information from all available sources uses SBAR, call-outs, check-backs and handoff techniques						

Use the following ratings. Remember, you are not describing an expert team, you are describing a student team.

Poor: Multiple critical behaviors absent or not performed well.
Average: Most behaviors present and adequately performed.
Excellent: All critical behaviors present and performed well.

© University of Washington Center for Health Sciences Interprofessional Education, Research & Practice
Last updated: February 22, 2017

Fig. 3. Performance Assessment of Communication and Teamwork–Novice Tool.

is utilized on occasion in acute care settings, such as in stroke treatment, health care teams primarily interact with patients at the bedside. Even though ECLIPSE faculties were aware that conducting the acute-care ECLIPSE simulations virtually would negatively affect the realism of the setting and expected outcomes, they decided to move forward anyway with web-based simulations because the value of the program had been evaluated so positively on the SET-M by students. The alternative was to cancel the ECLIPSE program for the academic year and deny 800 students a valuable IPE experience.

The TLC faculties planned for months for every imaginable contingency in the transition from in-person to web-based simulations conducted on a videoconference platform. With over 800 students' learning at stake, the extensive planning was time well spent because very few issues arose that were not anticipated in advance. However, student feedback indicated that a 3-hour Zoom meeting is too long without a break, which had not been included in the initial web-based simulations. In the in-person setting, if students needed a break, they could slip away from the simulation laboratory and come right back without their absence being noticed. On Zoom, when one student turned off his/her camera, others tended to follow suit, and then moderators suspected students were not engaged in their simulation.

The ECLIPSE transition experience demonstrated that web-based interprofessional simulations offer a comparable experience and a viable alternative when logistical challenges prevent in-person simulations. Web-based interprofessional collaborative practice simulations may work equally in-person simulations for students with more real-world clinical experience.[14] That is, students who have a more sophisticated understanding of authentic clinical contexts where interprofessional activities are carried out may be able to focus more effectively on interprofessional concepts during a web-

Table 2
PACT scores outcomes—Excellence in Interprofessional Simulation Education in-person and virtual sims comparison

Domains	In-Person Mean Scores	Virtual Mean Scores	Changes
Team structure	4.52	4.32	−0.20
Leadership	4.82	4.77	−0.05
Situational monitoring	4.34	4.09	−0.25
Mutual support	4.53	4.29	−0.24
Communication	4.46	4.29	−0.17
Overall mean	4.53	4.35	−0.18
Overall median	4.52	4.32	−0.20

5 = Excellent, 3 = Average, and 1 = Poor.

based experience than their peers with less clinical experience. More research is needed to explore the effectiveness of in-person versus web-based interprofessional simulation for students with different levels of clinical experience.

The ECLIPSE simulation program is now a well-established IPE program that has grown in both scope and excellence in the first 10 years, and it continues to gain momentum. The web-based simulation experiences lay the foundation for future virtual or hybrid models. Development is underway to extend existing acute-care simulation cases to ambulatory setting patient scenarios to accommodate the learning needs of students who will practice primarily in ambulatory settings. Extending existing acute care cases to follow-up care scenarios allows for transitional collaboration between learners as well. Additional plans for simulation development include the utilization of an existing educational electronic medical record (EMR) system for ECLIPSE-simulated patients. The proposed mock EMR mirrors the one used by the medical center affiliated with the university. The biggest barrier to implementing the mock EMR is cost (to be shared by all health care programs participating in the simulation), but if that barrier is overcome, the mock EMR will replace existing simulated paper patient charts and contribute to the realism of the simulation experiences.

Future interprofessional simulations may also take place within virtual reality (VR) spaces. As VR technology gains momentum in higher education, it will soon become possible for students to interact with those from other professions while at home in a headset. VR overcomes the logistical challenges of IPE while creating realism that closely mimics in-person simulations.

SUMMARY

When factors, such as scheduling, physical location, and interruptions in normal academic practice jeopardize in-person interprofessional simulation experiences, web-based interprofessional simulations offer opportunities to preserve continuity in IPE while meeting curricular requirements imposed by accreditors and other organizations that regulate academic health care education. The ECLISPE simulation was originally envisioned, designed, and facilitated by a committee consisting of faculty representatives from multiple health care professions, and the web-based version provided continuity in IPE despite barriers presented by a global pandemic. By expanding ECLIPSE to a web-based format, the ECLIPSE faculty team demonstrated that health care students can be prepared for interprofessional practice in a rapidly evolving health care environment even when time and space present barriers to interprofessional simulation.

The ECLIPSE faculty team continues to meet regularly to discuss all aspects of the simulation, analyze student evaluations, and review, adjust, and continuously improve the ECLIPSE experience. Implementing quality interprofessional simulations facilitates student achievement of interprofessional collaborative competencies, whether the simulations are delivered in person or online. As technology advances to make simulation environments more realistic, web-based interprofessional simulations will become even more effective and feasible alternatives to in-person simulations and support the development of practice-ready health care professionals.

CLINICS CARE POINTS

- Explore various teleconferencing platforms and other technology to find the best fit for the web-based simulation. Consider functionality, system reliability, customization, available support, and cost.

- Orient simulation faculty thoroughly to the web-based simulation platform to ensure sufficient understanding of technological features, functions, and limitations and how they may affect the simulation.

- Create roles and corresponding duties for faculty and staff who facilitate the activity.

- Conduct at least one dress-rehearsal simulation for all nonstudent participants before events involving students. Test all web-conferencing features and other technology that will be used during the simulation.

- Collect feedback from facilitators, students, and standardized patients for each simulation and make adjustments as necessary to ensure continuous improvement.

DISCLOSURE

The authors have nothing to disclose.

REFERENCES

1. Framework for action on Interprofessional Education and collaborative practice. World Health Organization. 1970. Available at: https://apps.who.int/iris/handle/10665/70185. Accessed February 23, 2022.
2. Core Competencies for Interprofessional Collaborative Practice: 2016 Update. https://ipec.memberclicks.net/assets/2016-Update.pdf. Accessed March 1, 2022.
3. About Us. Available at: https://www.ipecollaborative.org/about-us. Accessed February 23, 2022.
4. Aldriwesh MG, Alyousif SM, Alharbi NS. Undergraduate-level teaching and learning approaches for interprofessional education in the health professions: a systematic review. BMC Med Educ 2022;22(1):13.
5. Al-Jayyousi GF, Abdul Rahim H, Alsayed Hassan D, et al. Following interprofessional education: health education students' experience in a primary interprofessional care setting. J Multidiscip Healthc 2021;14:3253–65.
6. The New AACN Essentials. Available at: https://www.aacnnursing.org/AACN-Essentials. Accessed February 23, 2022.

7. Yune SJ, Park KH, Min YH, et al. Perceptions of the interprofessional education of the faculty and the level of interprofessional education competence of the students perceived by the faculty: a comparative study of medicine, nursing, and pharmacy. Korean J Med Educ 2020;32(1):23–33.

8. Lempicki KA, Holland CS. Web-based versus face-to-face interprofessional team encounters with standardized patients. Curr Pharm Teach Learn 2018;10(3): 344–51.

9. Cucinotta D, Vanelli M. WHO declares COVID-19 a Pandemic. Acta Biomed 2020;91(1):157–60.

10. Jones TA, Vidal G, Taylor C. Interprofessional education during the COVID-19 pandemic: finding the good in a bad situation. J Interprof Care 2020;34(5): 633–46.

11. About TeamSTEPPS. Available at: https://www.ahrq.gov/teamstepps/about-teamstepps/index.html. Accessed February 23, 2022.

12. Training guide: using simulation in TeamSTEPPS training. Available at: https://www.ahrq.gov/teamstepps/simulation/index.html. Accessed February 23, 2022.

13. Leighton K, Ravert P, Mudra V, et al. Updating the simulation effectiveness tool: item modifications and reevaluation of psychometric properties. Nurs Educ Perspect 2015;36(5):317–23.

14. Erlinger LR, Bartlett A, Perez A. High-fidelity mannequin simulation versus virtual simulation for recognition of critical events by student registered nurse anesthetists. AANA J 2019;87(2):105–9.

Innovative Pedagogical Approaches to Teaching Advanced Forensic Nursing

Patricia M. Speck, DNSc, FNP-BC, AFN-C, DF-IAFN, FAAFS, DF-AFN, FAAN,[a],*,
Elizabeth Burgess Dowdell, PhD, RN, AFN-C, FAAN[b],
Stacey A. Mitchell, DNP, MBA, MEd, RN, AFN-C, SANE-A, SANE-P, DF-AFN, FAAN[c]

KEYWORDS

- Forensic nursing • Death investigation • Forensic nursing certification
- Forensic nursing education • Social determinants of health
- Trauma health outcomes • Trauma-informed care • Vulnerable populations

KEY POINTS

- Violence and the subsequent trauma result in chronic disease affecting the lifespans of vulnerable populations, negatively influencing social determinants of health.
- Forensic nursing became a specialty in 1995, eventually giving rise to standardized graduate programs and Forensic Nursing Certification Board (FNCB) certification for the Generalist and Advanced Forensic Nurse.
- Past forensic nursing education emphasized psycho-motor skills in simulation labs, and most forensic nursing clinical experiences were observational only.
- Current approaches to teaching forensic nursing use virtual platforms, group work, interactive decisions, virtual case studies, and media to educate future advanced forensic nursing leaders.

BACKGROUND

Violence and the subsequent trauma outcomes result in chronic disease, affecting the lifespans of vulnerable populations.[1-3] Other variables having associations with poor health outcomes include racial or ethnic minority, socioeconomic disadvantage, and a diagnosis of certain medical, physical, or mental health conditions.[3-6] Epidemiologic studies provide insight into one vulnerable population—victims of crime.[7-9] The data are derived from police reports, crime reports, and other government agencies that

[a] Advanced Forensic Nursing, Department of Family, Community, & Health Systems, UAB | The University of Alabama at Birmingham School of Nursing, 1720 Second Avenue South, Birmingham, AL 35294-1210, USA; [b] Undergraduate Research, Villanova University, M. Louise Fitzpatrick College of Nursing, Driscoll Hall #326, 800 East, Lancaster Avenue, Villanova, PA 19085, USA; [c] Center of Excellence in Forensic Nursing, Texas A&M University Health Science Center, 8441 Riverside Parkway, Bryan, TX 77807, USA
* Corresponding author.
E-mail address: pmspeck@uab.edu

Nurs Clin N Am 57 (2022) 653–670
https://doi.org/10.1016/j.cnur.2022.07.004
0029-6465/22/© 2022 Elsevier Inc. All rights reserved.
nursing.theclinics.com

collect data.[10–12] Social determinants of health help health care providers understand disparities, provide a foundation in understanding risk and health trajectories, and underpin principles of trauma-informed care necessary for nurses[13] to reach and provide primary, secondary, and tertiary care for vulnerable populations.[3,14] Responding to disparities in health care, researchers use the social determinants of health to study stress-related diseases associated with a lifetime of trauma.[1,3–6,15] The inevitable growth of forensic nursing is directly related to increasing violence globally.

History of Forensic Nursing

The Latin word for nurture and sustenance of infants is *nurse*,[16] found in medicine and forensic medicine writings as old as 6000 years in China and Mesopotamia.[17] By the middle ages, Emmeline la Duchesse, a nurse matron, deaconess, documented victims of violence and testified about rape routinely in formal court records.[18,19] In the early 1800s, the Irish Sisters of Mercy spread the concept of *Careful Nursing*.[20] *Careful Nursing* is a model of respect for the innate dignity of the human condition,[21] and "a 'perfect' skill in fostering safety and comfort"[22] (p. 99), aligning with trauma-informed care.[13] Sr. Clare Moore, a Sisters of Mercy nun, influenced Florence Nightingale's memoirs that chronicle *Careful Nursing,* a testament to the influence of their friendship. Paralleling forensic nursing roles caring for victims of violence today, the Nightingale memoirs about caring for victims of the Crimea war contradict other autobiographies (such as Mary Jane Seacole) about the struggles between nursing groups during the period.[21–24] The cultural and racial conflicts persist today.[23–25] Following the Crimea war and into the late 1800s, a progressive understanding of psychiatric disorders grew as housing institutions for impoverished patients with mental health issues were exposed to be akin to prisons and poorhouses.[26] Hospitalization became the preferred and progressive treatment of the mentally insane, where patients received care from nurse deaconesses or matrons trained in *Careful Nursing*. The training incorporated higher education for these nurses who viewed nursing as both a science and an art.[21,22] In the early 1900s, nurses were also activists, and psychiatric nurses joined the asylum workers union to help transform the institutional asylum system.[27] These early psychiatric-mental health nurses and corrections caretakers formed the historical basis for those who are now known as forensic nurses. The role of the forensic nurse is important to understand as the development of community opportunities facilitates a unique path in nursing, which is different from hospital nursing.

Evolution of Forensic Nursing Education

Over the twentieth century, nurses expanded into several patient care settings through public health and community nursing, integrating forensic nursing principles with populations vulnerable to poverty, crime, and violence.[28,29] These community patients came from migrant populations living in squalor conditions in large cities. The populations experiencing poverty and starvation (now known as social determinants of health) turned to crime, which resulted in the intersection of corrections and psychiatric-mental health nursing. The stress resulted in interpersonal (dating, workplace, technology) and family violence (child, elder, domestic), as well as other types of violence, which are all areas of forensic nursing practice today. As understanding of trauma and vulnerable populations increased, the forensic nursing role was continuously refined, and in 1992, Virginia Lynch, MSN, RN, conceptualized a theoretic framework for the practice of the forensic nurse in the United States.[30] By 1995, the American Nurses Association recognized forensic nursing as a specialty, and subsequently, there was a proliferation of graduate programs in forensic nursing. Initially, the programs were distinctive, reflecting the expertise of the lead faculty. Students expected the graduate education to reflect the continuing education in forensic nursing with content siloed in subspecialties (such as sexual assault, domestic violence, forensic psychology, corrections, forensic science and others), and similar to continuing education offered by professional organizations. Consequently, one subspecialty, sexual assault nurse examiners (SANE), gained notoriety and considerable funding to the detriment of other areas in forensic nursing.

The death investigator role is a subspecialty role in forensic nursing,[31] and passionate forensic nurses gained skills and developed practices in death investigation outside the forensic nursing professional organizations. Historically taught in continuing education courses and seminars, the investigation of death is becoming increasingly complex, partially because of the COVID-19 global pandemic, but also because of the aging baby boomer population that is living longer with chronic health issues. Forensic nurse death investigators bring knowledge to interprofessional teams about disease and disease progression, pharmacology, and the normal aging processes.[31] They examine decedents and scenes using a medical lens to determine if the death is suspicious. The role of the forensic nurse death investigator demands detailed, documented observations which are assembled by the medical examiner or coroner who has the ultimate responsibility for determining the cause and manner of death. Expanding practice roles of the advanced forensic nurse allow for Certified Registered Nurse Practitioners (CRNPs) in some states to sign the death certificate,[32] sometimes limited to cases where deaths are due to natural causes or there is a contracted relationship with the CRNP, such as in palliative care.

At the start of the millennium, forensic nursing educators met to frame the practice domains and performance measures in graduate nursing education.[33] Building on the 2004 and 2014 educator meetings, the Forensic Nursing Certification Board (FNCB) completed a Delphi study with qualitative analysis in 2020 to 21. The results from the Delphi study provided the basis for standardization necessary to offer comprehensive certification for the Generalist and Advanced Forensic Nurse.[34] AACN *Essentials* for Level 1 and 2 nursing education[35] guided the work of the FNCB. The graduate-prepared forensic nurse today is a specialist nurse with specific forensic nursing knowledge in three pillars of science: legal principles, forensic science, and forensic nursing science. Forensic nursing practice is person-centered, trauma-informed, based in quality and safety, professionalism, technology, population care, and lifelong learning, leadership, and professionalism, and aligns with the *Essentials* educational core competencies guiding the nursing profession.[34]

The challenge for forensic nursing educators in teaching unique, subspecialty knowledge is pivoting away from traditional classroom instruction and face-to-face simulation laboratory exercises toward contemporary, evidence-based models of authentic, technology-supported learning in alignment with the nursing and FNCB core competencies. The pivot also includes integrating technology effectively to meet all levels of learning in the future. The expectation is that faculty guide students' exploration of knowledge, helping them look for connectedness and associations in their explanations, by using an innovative design to achieve "learning outcomes and operational principles"[36] (p. 13), an expectation in graduate education specialty training. During the COVID-19 pandemic, learning theories provided guidance in the integration of innovative virtual technology into forensic nursing curriculum. These technological approaches in pedagogy align with nursing and forensic nursing core competencies (domains), descriptions of practice, context for practice, and performance measures for the unique content necessary for generalist and advanced forensic nursing practices globally.[34] Learning theory underpins evidence-based teaching innovation to engage students in advanced forensic nursing activities in technologically supported learning environments.

CONTEMPORARY FORENSIC NURSING EDUCATION

Learning theory is under continuous development and guides educators by providing models for learning outcomes.[36,37] More complex is the recent challenge of threading core competencies from professional nursing organizations guiding nursing education documents.[38–41] Online courses in pre-COVID-19 conceptual designs[42] generate instructional design limitations in the classroom, and a preference by some faculty for face-to-face learning.[43] In forensic nursing, providers of continuing education simulation taught specific psycho-motor skills in face-to-face simulation labs[44–47] using the "see-one, do-one, teach-one" method of acquiring skills. The simulation method was thought to be satisfactory as most forensic nursing clinical experiences were observational only, because of the likelihood of future adjudication. Students have potential to be an inexperienced naïve witness to the process, and there is a reluctance to involve students in any legally sensitive, authentic field experience in forensic nursing.

Critical Thinking Versus Creative Thinking

As in all nursing education, Bloom's taxonomy guides initial activities in forensic nursing education, with a view of the taxonomy as a hierarchy that reflects increasingly complex ways of thinking.[48,49] Over the last 20 years, revisions of Bloom's Taxonomy proposed two levels of learning, notably critical thinking, and creative thinking.[49] Nurse faculty often say, without understanding, that they are teaching *critical thinking*. Unfortunately, critical thinking evaluation captures a lower level of testable knowledge in forensic nursing, where *creative thinking* is more complex. The complexity often integrates concepts in designed circumstances and requires demonstration of learner approaches to include application of the same knowledge in a variety of forensic nursing situations. For the faculty, threading forensic nursing core competencies through an assigned creative thinking product is more difficult to assess, and more difficult to grade. For the purposes of exploring forensic nursing education, the adaptation and modifications in forensic nursing education reveal a pattern and order of thinking unique in forensic nursing practice and education, described in **Table 1**.

The global COVID-19 pandemic required re-thinking of educational approaches, and in many cases re-training of faculty in instructional technology. As such, there was a rapid integration of technology, beginning with online virtual and hybrid courses seeking to teach unique forensic nursing roles and activities to online graduate students. However, the technology revolution in coursework was often criticized by students who wanted more than a presentation of facts (also known as *Death by PowerPoint*), conceptual interrelationships between professional roles (also known as *multidisciplinary teams*), and procedures (also known as *skills and techniques*). All were one-dimensional and integrated into existing practices without complex and creative learning outcomes. The only basis faculty had for course improvement was student feedback, and student feedback was not good. Student negativity was related to course instructions, content, relevancy, application to practice, and measurement of learning methods, which demanded new approaches.

The new way of thinking about learning in forensic nursing education created opportunity to not only apply learning theory, but to capture the creative thinking necessary to solve problems in real-world situations faced by today's generalist and advanced forensic nurse. Learning theory provides a framework for several dimensions of

Table 1
Modified Bloom's learning taxonomy for learning in forensic nursing

Learning Cognitive Categories (Basic to Complex)	Forensic Nursing Examples	General Technologies	Typical Key Words in Objectives/Goals
Remembering—Knowledge includes remembering, recognizing, recalling relevant knowledge from long-term memory.	Often forensic nurses recognize and recall from previous learning, such as definitions, facts or lists with an ability to verbally recite. An example is the Federal Rules of Evidence or the hypothalamic–pituitary–adrenal axis (HPA axis) with *little in-depth knowledge.*	Powerpoint presentations, electronic books, electronic flash cards, all helping identify, relate, list, define, repeat, and recognize repetition reading based on rote learning about topics of interest in forensic nursing.	Learning words associated with objectives and goals include acquire, defines, describes, identifies, knows, labels, lists, matches, memorize, name, outlines, recalls, recognizes, relates, repeat reproduces, selects, states.
Understanding—Comprehension includes grasp of meanings from oral, written, and graphic messages and includes interpreting, exemplifying, classifying, summarizing, inferring, comparing, and explaining.	Forensic nurses often construct *meaning myopically and are challenged to explain or show complex forensic nursing tasks.* For instance, teaching about trauma-informed care results in test score improvement through comprehension of new knowledge, exemplifying, classifying, summarizing, inferring, comparing, or explaining in the educational deliverables, for example, quizzes, paper, posters, presentations.	Cooperative learning helps forensic nurses understand difficult concepts from borrowed science through collaborative activities, for example, discussion boards, literature searches, and demonstration of integration of new knowledge. May include inter-professional and multi-disciplinary activities, coaching, mentoring, and self-reflection. Forensic nurses work in small groups (online) on assigned projects under faculty guidance who monitors teams, ensuring learners are on task, AND producing correct answers.	Learning words associated with objectives and goals include comprehends, conclude, converts, defends, describe, differentiate discuss, distinguishes, draw, estimates, explains, express, extends, generalizes, gives an example, identify, illustrate, infers, interprets, locates, paraphrases, predicts, recognize, report, represent, restate, review, review, rewrites, summarizes, translates

(continued on next page)

Table 1
(continued)

Learning Cognitive Categories (Basic to Complex)	Forensic Nursing Examples	General Technologies	Typical Key Words in Objectives/Goals
Applying—Application includes carrying out or using a procedure through execution or implementation in all practice settings, and includes the ability to use learned material, or to implement material in new and concrete situations, for example, where previous learning informs application.	For the forensic nurse, a demonstrative execution of competence is an example when applying protocols to situations, such as evidence collection, adjusting for patient preference (eg, person-centered care) throughout the process. For the forensic nurse, application of new learning requires analysis for outcome measurements, which is knowledge application, for example, trauma-informed practice changes where application is behaviorally driven.	In forensic nursing, technologies are useful in application and provide an opportunity for demonstration of the application. For instance, product development may include application of quality and safety tools detecting improvement or to situations where learned material is used through products like models, presentations, interviews, or simulations.	Learning words associated with objectives and goals include applies, calculates, changes, computes, constructs, employs, demonstrates, dramatizes, develops, discovers, exhibits, interprets, illustrates, manipulates, modifies, operates, organizes, practices, predicts, prepares, produces, relates, shows, solves, translates, uses.
Analyzing—Analysis includes the ability to break down or distinguish the parts of material into its components so that its organizational structure may be better understood and determining how the parts relate to one another or *determining new relationships* and to an overall structure or purpose.	For all forensic nurses, learning supporting the ability to analyze a situation or patient, determining how the parts relate, and is an essential skill. The skill can be as simple as troubleshooting an equipment failure, or as complex as the first step in quality improvement, recognizing fallacy in a situation.	The forensic nurse exercises mental actions, which include first questioning what happened, and they may run a test or investigate using root cause analysis. The analysis results in organizing distinguishing facts, differentiating, and attributing; to assist in the analysis, forensic nurses often use spreadsheets, surveys, charts, or diagrams, and graphic representations, for example, photographs of injury.	Learning words associated with objectives and goals include analyzes, attributing, breaks down, categorize, classify, compares, contrasts, deconstructs, deduce, detect, diagrams, differentiates, discriminates, dissect, distinguishes, examine, experiment, identifies, illustrates, infers, inquire, inspect, investigate, organizing, outlines, probe, relates, scrutinize, selects, separates, survey.

		Learning words associated with objectives and goals
Evaluating—Evaluation includes making judgments *according to circumstance and environment* based on criteria and standards through checking and critiquing, that reflects a forensic nurse ability to judge, check, and even critique the value of processes and materials for a given purpose.	The forensic nurse uses evaluation to put elements together to form a coherent or functional whole, such as justifying a request, or reorganizes elements into a new pattern or structure of thinking through a process of generating, planning, or producing new ways of thinking. Creating requires forensic nurses to put parts together in a new way or synthesizing mental thought parts into something new and different and is the most difficult mental function in the new learning taxonomy.	Learning words associated with objectives and goals include appraise, argue, assess, choose, compare, conclude, considers, contrast, criticize, critiques, decide, deduce, defends, describes discriminates, estimates, evaluate, explain, infer, interprets, judges, justifies, measures, rate, relates, select, summarizes, supports, validates, values.
Creating—Synthesis includes putting elements together to form a coherent or functional whole, *even if there is absent information* and reorganizing elements into a new pattern or structure through generating, planning, or producing with the ability to put parts together to form a coherent or unique new whole.	Making judgments based on criteria and forensic nursing and nursing standards through checking, re-checking, re-visiting, and critiquing. Critiques, recommendations, and reports are some of the products created to synthesize and show the dynamic formative and summative evaluative processes in forensic nursing. In the newer taxonomy, evaluating comes before creating as it is often a necessary part of the precursory behavior before one creates something. Examples of the creations	The forensic nurse creates new models of thinking in the implementation of systems change to new information, all while networking with technology in planning organization of structural patterns into coherent or new unique wholes, such as in the development of new program initiatives based in research outcomes. Nimbleness is an essential characteristic of the forensic nurse in practice who constantly implementing the nursing process of Assessment, Diagnosis, Planning, Learning words associated with objectives and goals include arrange, assemble, categorize, combine, collect, complies, compose, construct, creates, derive, design, develop, devises, documents, explains, formulate, generates, generalize, invent, modify, organize, originate, plan, prepare, predict, propose, rearranges, relates, reorganizes, revises, rewrites, set up, summarizes, tells, writes.

(continued on next page)

Table 1
(continued)

Learning Cognitive Categories (Basic to Complex)	Forensic Nursing Examples	General Technologies	Typical Key Words in Objectives/ Goals
	include determining priority in operations or process manuals, design apps to improve safety and health, or solve a problem or create a scientific opinion for the judicial processes (eg, testimony) in forensic nursing.	Intervention, and Evaluation (ADPIE) in unique practice settings.	

Adapted to demonstrate forensic nursing education from: Anderson, Krawthwohl, & Airasian, 2001; Bloom, Engelhart, Furst, & Krathwohl, 1956; Picciano, 2017.

knowledge necessary for complex learning in forensic nursing: factual, conceptual, procedural, and metacognitive. These dimensions are viewed through the lens of forensic nursing in **Table 2** with examples. By developing a model based on Bloom's revised taxonomy, a group of forensic nursing faculty created innovative approaches to teaching and learning across all knowledge dimensions specifically to show complexity in learning about forensic nursing practice and, in the demonstration case that follows, a death investigation.

INSTRUCTIONAL CASE STUDY

Faculty in a forensic nursing education program, who are the authors of the present article, design instruction using principles of team learning with strategies to solve an uncommon problem facing nurses in hospitals and in palliative care. Nurses often enter forensic nursing programs with the intent of running for election as their rural community's coroner position. Although faculty provided students with a smorgasbord of cases with children through the older adult, the description of the assignment module that follows serves as an introduction to the role of the forensic nurse death investigator, working as a coroner or in a medical examiner's office. The case is focused on an adult decedent found in a bathroom, a frequent discovery of hospital nurses and families, and provides clear examples of how technology supports student achievement of core competencies in forensic nursing at the highest levels of Bloom's taxonomy revisions.

The goal is to move students through a logically designed learning scenario that ends with metacognitive application of learning in the Death Certificate document. The case scenario involves the discovery of a patient on the bathroom floor by the nurse. The bathroom 360° video [https://youtu.be/fldQLFC2bLU?list=PL_kvth9t2749hPRsTzKvnUqvSw6FfiYJl] provides students with a view of the scene in all directions, and the scene still photographs [https://sway.office.com/GTgHxdv235IV0Dxs?ref=LinkNeed] provide additional, more detailed views. The student, when presented with the scenario, uses newly acquired knowledge to analyze and synthesize the facts and evaluate the information to deduce the probable *cause and manner of death* and document on the death certificate.

Module and Assessments

Virtual learning has multiple meanings. For the purposes of the course design, the authors use various deliverables to apply a variety of very flexible activities for learning in institutionally supported technologies, as noted in **Table 3**. With the assessment products for all levels of learning in mind, the faculty designed a module with specific instructions to first learn basic knowledge necessary for problem-solving. The items for teaching included library access to articles, media, and webinars. Faculty instructed students to begin with media, *FRONTLINE: Post Mortem—Death Investigation in America* [https://www.pbs.org/wgbh/pages/frontline/post-mortem/], to frame the problem.[50] The PBS website offers links to related programs, allowing students to build a toolbox of media resources for their community of forensic nurses.

Faculty advise students to use shared and institutionally supported software for team product development and synchronous collaboration (eg, Google Docs, MS Teams). Faculty are often invited to join student team meetings to contribute to the students' journey of discovery. A PowerPoint presentation by a subject matter expert with a decade of forensic nursing death investigation provides basic information in the form of definitions and explanations necessary for *knowledge* in the field. A synchronous Zoom meeting entitled *Candid Conversation with the Expert* follows, which is a

Table 2
Taxonomy of knowledge necessary for complex learning and thinking in forensic nursing

Taxonomy	Definition	Example
Factual Knowledge	Basic elements of the forensic nursing discipline, attempts to define, describe, and categorize (knowledge that is basic to forensic nursing). This dimension refers to essential facts, terminology, details, or elements students must know or be familiar with in order to understand the forensic nursing discipline or solve a problem in it.	What exists in the three pillars (legal principles, forensic science, and forensic nursing) defining the practices of forensic nurses?
Conceptual Knowledge	Looks for causality and correlation, and work with variables in relationships with the patient, community, and systems (knowledge of classifications, principles, generalizations, forensic nursing theories, models of practice, or structures pertinent to forensic nursing.).	Why does this happen in the context of forensic nursing practices?
Procedural Knowledge	Describes interventions for teaching targeted outcomes and operational principles in forensic nursing practice (refers to information or knowledge that helps students to do something specific to a discipline, subject, or area of study. It also refers to methods of inquiry, very specific or finite skills, algorithms, techniques, and particular methodologies.).	How do I achieve this outcome in forensic nursing interventions?
Metacognitive Knowledge	The awareness of one's own cognition and particular cognitive processes. It is strategic or reflective knowledge about how to go about solving problems, cognitive tasks, to include contextual and conditional knowledge and knowledge of self and personal learning methods.	What knowledge and resources do forensic nurses use to solve the problem to create an optimal outcome for patients, communities, and systems?

Adapted From: Anderson LW, Krawthwohl DR, Airasian PW, et al., 2001; Wilson 2005.

Table 3
Learning level, death investigation course deliverables, and technology use in the module design

Learning Levels	Death Investigation Course Deliverables	Technology Use
Knowledge	PBS Frontline viewing Presentation by subject matter expert Interactive online course Evidence for forensic nursing role	Media Power point Computer Library services
Understanding	Graded discussion board with rubric conceptualizing the patient and family using previous learning from last term understanding there is a process for notification	Canvas Learning management system
Applying	Graded discussion board with rubric that formalizes thoughts and associations, and mandates replies that have specific content defined in the application of new knowledge	Canvas Learning management system
Analyzing	Graded team discussion with rubric that mandates associations and the logic necessary with an evidence-base, provided in the reading materials with an option to find unique resources for relationships in information	Electronic library resources PDFs Search engines, for example, CINHAL, PubMed, Scopus
Evaluation	Team member engagement with rubric recording that follows the analysis of the knowledge and application of knowledge to case. Student-led module evaluation Quiz	Go React Kaltura recording Just in Time survey Canvas Question Bank Quiz (Respondus LockDown Browser)
Creating	Team assimilation of facts presented in photographs with evidence of logic from deliverables above with probable cause and manner of death	Completion of electronic AL Death Certificate

synchronous opportunity for students to engage with an actual forensic nurse with expertise in death investigation. With specific articles addressing the knowledge base and forensic nursing role, the online resources to guide new knowledge acquisition (eg, Census data, CDC's Social Determinants of Health, Morbidity and Mortality reports), students are ready to begin assimilating new knowledge for analysis of the evidence base through asynchronous graded discussions. The discussions are carried out on the discussion board in the institution's learning management system and guided by a rubric with criteria covering key elements in determination of *cause and manner of death*. They evaluate their peers' posts through their structured asynchronous replies, pointing out missing key elements and integrating the absent key elements into the learning process. By the end of the graded discussion board assignment, students show the first four domains of learning according to Bloom's taxonomy—knowledge, understanding, applying, and analyzing.

To promote higher levels of learning in evaluation and metacognitive creations, the course design uses 360° photographic technology to provide realistic details about the case, and a structured rubric is used to guide demonstration of metacognitive learning. The assumption by faculty is that students taking the Death Investigation module have access to and will use previous course resources in their electronic tool-boxes. Faculty use the quiz tool in their learning management system to assess the student's knowledge retention from previous learning and acquisition of new knowledge. Faculty also ask students to evaluate the course design and teaching strategies using Just in Time questions in a survey tool for future course improvement. Faculty use Go React with Kaltura (video assessment software) to record discussions about the evaluation of the case and the possibilities not shown in the information provided about the decedent discovery. The discussions emphasize conceptual evaluation and creative thinkingin the construction of new explanations derived from evidence in the photographic record of the setting and the staged evidence in the bathroom, demonstrating the higher two domains of learningaccording to Blooms's taxonomy - evalutting and creating. Faculty remain available to students to explain the intentions of the representations in the photographic evidence and compensate for the limitations of moulage, acknowledging the impossibility of recreating a real death scene.

Planning for the photographic technology and staging the simulation scenes required significant coordination working with the school of nursing's Instructional Design and Simulation faculty to create realistic simulations by using moulage on mannequins. Once a death scene like that often encountered by forensic nurses was set up, the entire room, staged bathroom, and the draped mannequin were filmed and photographed using 360° photographic technology. The technologies and web sites faculty used in the implementation of the Death Investigation module are listed in **Table 4**.

The Death Investigation module is structured as a 2-week endeavor for graduate students who spend an average of 12 to 15 hours each week in forensic nursing specialty coursework. There are multiple steps and several deliverables for

Table 4
Technology to facilitate graduate forensic nursing student learning about death investigation

Technology Name	Description	Web Location
Canvas	Learning Management System	Canvas
Just in Time	Survey platform	Qualtrics
360° photography and photographs	Provides a comprehensive view of a space	UAB SON Instructional Design department
Kaltura	Recording software	Kaltura Video Hub
GoReact	Video assessment tool with opportunity for immediate feedback	Go React
Respondus LockDown Browser	Proctoring software for quizzes	Respondus LockDown Browswer
Zoom	Video conferencing	Zoom
MicroSoft Teams	Meeting software and synchronous document activity	MS TEAMS
Google Docs	Synchronous document activity	Google Docs
Internet sites, for example, CDC, Census data, Morbidity and Mortality	Facilitates access to morbidity and mortality data necessary to understand population burden and social determinants of health	CDC Social Determinants of Health AND United States Census AND Morbidity and Mortality Reports – Deaths

Note: the technology listed is not an endorsement, but a reflection of available institutional technologies to faculty at the University of Alabama at Birmingham School of Nursing.

Table 5
Death investigation grading rubric

Discussion Topic	5 of 100 Points	Description Expectations	Sources of Information
Community Description	2	Identify community population with 5 characteristics (population, income, morbidity/mortality, crime stats, etc.)	*US Census Fact Finder (Links to an external site.)* *2018 Crime in the US (Links to an external site.)* Other sources found by teams
Family Members	0.75	Complete Genogram for the decedent who may have parents, grandparents, siblings, children, describing gender, age, relationship. For 3 family members, describe traumatic life experiences	Use Smart Art in Word - Hierarchy Attach to graded DB
Family Informant	0.25	Write subjective information provided by informant in their voice; quotes are objective	Use scenarios created from NFN 622 Advanced Forensic Nursing I course (Fall) to inform your family
Visible Evidence	1	All simulations are potential crime scenes; begin the description of the scene and move inward using learning over 2 terms	Cite references for assertions about evidence (copy and paste from previous modules and course deliverables)
Possible Cause & Manner of Death	1	Discuss all possible differential diagnoses for cause and manner of death. Your team's logic matters here! Transfer all information to the Death Certificate	The graded DB should have all possible differentials for cause and manner of death. Deposit the completed Death Certificate with logical cause and manner of death

students to complete in the Death Investigation module. The final assessment product is a complex evaluation, submitted by students as an electronic death certificate, created usingdecadent's information to document Bloom's higher domains of learning to evaluate the scenario and create the logical *cause and manner of death*. A detailed grading rubric (**Table 5**) and clear, concise student instructions to complete the assignment are essential.

The death certificate (**Fig. 1**) is the final submission in the module, showing student achievement of metacognitive, creative learning.

RESULTS

Student responses to course evaluation surveys were positive and included, "I am a palliative care nurse and needed this module years ago!" and "I loved working with

Fig. 1. Alabama death certificate.

my team brainstorming possible causes of death with case we chose." Suggested changes, such as "I need rapid technology support for the required assignments in the course," have been incorporated with a *Quick Links* section that includes technical support resources and increasing clarity in instructions over the years.

By the end of the module, students have gained required knowledge and skills through creative learning to successfully complete a death certificate, an essential skill necessary for the advanced forensic nurse responsible for care of patients in organizations. Mastery of the skill ensures efficient collection of accurate death data for morbidity and mortality records. Representing available facts accurately on a death certificate requires attainment of knowledge at all levels of Bloom's taxonomy. Knowledge acquisition and assessment of learning are supported by selection of appropriately aligned learning technologies.

SUMMARY

Educational technology available today supports interactive group decision-making, team collaboration, and media-enhanced case studies to teach forensic nurses about death investigation. Continuous advances in technology hold great potential to enhance innovation in education for the future advanced forensic nursing leaders. With the advent of forensic nursing core competencies, descriptions and context for forensic nursing practices, and content for robust forensic nursing curriculum, graduate forensic nursing educators have the opportunity to align curricula with general nursing education core competencies for forensic nursing instruction.

In the Death Investigation module, using a purposeful design and readily available technology, faculty delivered evidence-based instruction unique to the forensic nursing discipline. Online delivery of complex conceptual forensic nursing knowledge facilitated by use of video and image recording technology to standardize student experiences, discussions, and procedural knowledge create an instructional strategy to challenge students with expectations of metacognitive complexity to determine the cause and manner of death. Problem-solving of complex tasks by applying metacognitive processes that include knowledge of self and abilities results in a successful learning design for students in graduate forensic nursing coursework. The assignment module described in the article has potential for replication in other forensic nursing programs and makes possible measurement of all knowledge dimensions in generalist and advanced forensic nursing practices.

CLINICS CARE POINTS

- Correctly completed death certificates are the foundation for morbidity and mortality reports.
- The Future of Nursing 2020 to 2030 supports expansion of nursing practices such as the completion of death certificates by nurses caring for known patients.
- Learning technologies play a key role in supporting interactive learning, student engagement, and authentic assessment in forensic nursing topics.
- Forensic nursing subspecialties include coroners and death investigators.
- Generalist and Advanced Forensic Nurses are essential members of health care teams addressing violence and trauma outcomes.

ACKNOWLEDGMENTS

UAB SON Instructional Design: Matthew Jennings, Director, James Clark, and James Henson; UAB SON Clinical Simulation Lab: Drs Penni Watts, Director, and Tracie White, and Ms. Caroline Cartledge.

DISCLOSURE

Drs P.M. Speck, E.B. Dowdell, and S.A. Mitchell serve as Board members of the Forensic Nursing Certification Board (FNCB), a nonprofit promoting evidence-based forensic nursing certifications. They have no other disclosures that affect the content in the submitted publication.

REFERENCES

1. McCollum D. COLEVA — Consequences of lifetime exposure to violence and Abuse 2009. Available at: https://www.avahealth.org/file_download/inline/f89d58b2-1371-40a4-99c9-c4d2309eedf0. Accessed January 11, 2022.
2. Rural Health Information Hub. Social determinants of health for rural people. 2020-22. Available at: https://www.ruralhealthinfo.org/topics/social-determinants-of-health#rural-difference. Accessed January 11, 2022.
3. Office of Disease Prevention and Health Promotion. Social determinants of health. Healthy people 2020 2021, December 21. Available at: https://www.healthypeople.gov/2020/topics-objectives/topic/social-determinants-of-health. Accessed January 10, 2022.
4. Picard M, McEwen BS. Psychological Stress and Mitochondria: A Conceptual Framework. Psychosom Med 2018;80(2):126–40.
5. Jones CW, Esteves KC, Gray SAO, et al. The transgenerational transmission of maternal adverse childhood experiences (ACEs): Insights from placental aging and infant autonomic nervous system reactivity. Psychoneuroendocrinology 2019;106:20–7.
6. Seal SV, Turner JD. The 'Jekyll and Hyde' of Gluconeogenesis: Early Life Adversity, Later Life Stress, and Metabolic Disturbances. Int J Mol Sci 2021;22(7):3344.
7. World Health Organization. Global status report on preventing violence against children. 2020.
8. Richmond TS, Foman M. Firearm Violence: A Global Priority for Nursing Science. J Nurs Scholarsh 2019;51(3):229–40.
9. United Nations. A New Era of Conflict and Violence. Available at: https://www.un.org/sites/un2.un.org/files/un75_conflict_violence.pdf. Accessed January 11, 2022.
10. U S Department of Health and Human Services. Community Violence Prevention. Violence Prevention n.d. Available at: https://www.cdc.gov/violenceprevention/communityviolence/. Accessec January 11, 2022.
11. World Health Organization. First ever Global Report on Violence and Health released: new WHO report presents more complete picture of global violence. Geneva (Switzerland): World Health Organization; 2002.
12. World Health Organization. World report on violence and health: Summary. Geneva (Switzerland): World Health Organization; 2002. p. 54.
13. Dowdell, E.B. and P.M. Speck, Foundations For Trauma Informed Care in Nursing Practice. American Journal of Nursing, 2022. 122(4).
14. World Health Organization. Violence and injury prevention and disability: Global campaign for violence prevention. [Internet]. Available at: http://www.who.int/

violence_injury_prevention/violence/global_campaign/en/index.html.   Accessed January 11, 2022.

15. Selye H. Stress without Distress. Philadelphia: Lippincott; 1974.
16. Harper, D., Etymology of nurse, in Online Etymology Dictionary. n.d., Douglas Harper.
17. Payne-James J. History and development of forensic medicine and pathology. Forensic Medicine: Clinical and Pathological Aspects 2003;3–12.
18. Cumston CG. Note on the History of Forensic Medicine of the Middle Ages. J Crim Law Criminol 1913;3(6):855.
19. Shahar S. Fourth estate: a history of women in the middle ages. United Kingdom: Routledge Taylor & Francis Group; 1983. p. 390.
20. Paradis MR, Hart EM, O'Brien MJ. The Sisters of Mercy in the Crimean War: Lessons for Catholic health care. Linacre Q 2017;84(1):29–43.
21. Meehan TC. The Careful Nursing philosophy and professional practice model. J Clin Nurs 2012;21(19–20):2905–16.
22. Meehan TC. Careful nursing: A model for contemporary nursing practice. J Adv Nurs 2003;44(1):99–107.
23. Nagai K. Florence Nightingale and the Irish uncanny. Feminist Rev 2004;(77): 26–45.
24. Seacole M. Wonderful Adventures of Mrs Seacole in many Lands. London: James Blackwood; 1857.
25. Santos FBO, Rabelo ARM, França BD, et al. Black women in nursing history: the cultural competence in Maria Barbosa Fernandes' trajectory. Revista brasileira de enfermagem 2020;73(suppl 4):e20190221.
26. Bartlett P. The Asylum, the Workhouse, and the Voice of the Insane Poor in 19th-Century England. Int J Law Psychiatry 1998;21(4):421–32.
27. Nolan PW. A history of the training of asylum nurses. J Adv Nurs 1993;18(8): 1193–201.
28. Ruel SR. Lillian Wald: a pioneer of home health care in the United States. Home Healthc Nurse 2014;32(10):597–600.
29. Silverstein NG. Lillian Wald at Henry Street, 1893-1895. ANS Adv Nurs Sci 1985; 7(2):1–12.
30. Lynch, V. A., Clinical forensic nursing: A descriptive study in role development [Advisor: Janet Barber-Duval; Thesis, University of Texas Arlington. Arlington, TX, 1991.
31. Drake SA, Tabor P, Hamilton H, et al. Nurses and Medicolegal Death Investigation. J forensic Nurs 2020;16(4):207–14.
32. Alabama Board of Nursing. FAQs-Practice-Advanced Practice-CRNP-What can CRNPs and CNMs sign for in Alabama?. Available at: https://www.abn.alabama.gov/faqs/#faq/what-can-crnps-and-cnms-sign-for-in-alabama.   Accessed January 11, 2022.
33. Education Committee. Core Competencies for the Advanced Practice Forensic Nursing, 2004. 2004, October. Available at: https://cdn.ymaws.com/www.forensicnurses.org/resource/resmgr/Education/APN_Core_Curriculum_Document.pdf. Accessed January 11, 2022.
34. Speck, P.M. Aligning forensic nursing pedagogy and practice [Poster]. in 2021 Health Policy Conference. 2021, September. Washington, DC: American Academy of Nursing, October 8, 2021.
35. American Association of Colleges of Nursing. Re-Envisioning the AACN essentials: Frequently asked questions 2021. Available at: https://www.aacnnursing.

org/Portals/42/Downloads/Essentials/Essentials-Revision-Frequently-Asked-Questions.pdf. Accessed January 11, 2022.

36. Graham CR, Henrie CR, Gibbons AS. Developing models and theory for blended learning researc, In Blended learning. Research perspectives 2013;2:13–33.

37. Wilson LO. Anderson and Krathwohl Bloom's Taxonomy Revised: Understanding the New Version of Bloom's Taxonomy. 2016, 2013, 2005, 2001. Available at: https://quincycollege.edu/wp-content/uploads/Anderson-and-Krathwohl_Revised-Blooms-Taxonomy.pdf. Accessed January 11, 2022.

38. American Association of Colleges of Nursing. The Essentials: Core Competencies for Professional Nursing Education 2021 May 5, 2021. Available at: https://www.aacnnursing.org/Portals/42/AcademicNursing/pdf/Essentials-2021.pdf. Accessed January 11, 2022.

39. American Association of Colleges of Nursing. The essentials of Baccalaureate education for professional nursing practice. Washington, DC: American Association of Colleges of Nursing; 1998.

40. American Association of Colleges of Nursing. The essentials of Doctoral education for advanced nursing practice, 28. Washington, DC: American Association of Colleges of Nursing; 2006.

41. American Association of Colleges of Nursing. The essentials of Masters education in nursing practice. Washington, DC: American Association of Colleges of Nursing AACN; 2011.

42. Baron KA. Changing to Concept-Based Curricula: The Process for Nurse Educators. Open Nurs J 2017;11:277–87.

43. Paul J, Jefferson F. A Comparative Analysis of Student Performance in an Online vs. Face-to-Face Environmental Science Course From 2009 to 2016. Front Computer Sci 2019;1.

44. Baker J, Kelly PJ, Carlson K, et al. SANE-A-PALOOZA: Logistical Development and Implementation of a Clinical Immersion Course for Sexual Assault Nurse Examiners. J forensic Nurs 2016;12(4):176–82.

45. Ferguson C, Faugno D. The SAFE CARE model: Maintaining competency in sexual assault examinations utilizing patient simulation methods. J forensic Nurs 2009;5(2):109–14.

46. Mahoney G. Competency assessment in sexual assault nursing practice: an evidence-based Approach. Ann Arbor, MI: ProQuest Dissertations Publishing; 2012.

47. Mitchell SA, Charles L, Downing N. Increasing Access to Forensic Nursing Services in Rural and Under-Served Areas of Texas. J Forensic Nurs 2021;18(1):21–9.

48. Bloom BS, Engelhart MD, Furst EJ, et al. Taxonomy of Educational Objectives. Handbook I: The Cognitive Domain. In: Bloom BS, editor. New York: David McKay Company, Inc; 1956.

49. Anderson LW, Krawthwohl DR, Airasian PW, et al. A taxonomy for learning, teaching, and assessing: a revision of Bloom's taxonomy of educational Objectives. New York: Pearson, Allyn & Bacon; 2001. Accessed January 11, 2022.

50. Frontline: Post Mortem Death Investigation in America. Corporation for Public Broadcasting. Available at: https://www.pbs.org/wgbh/pages/frontline/post-mortem/.

Nursing Students with Disabilities

A Guide to Providing Accommodations

Laura Stinnette Lucas, DNP, APRN-CNS, RNC-OB, C-EFM*,
JoAnne Silbert-Flagg, DNP, CPNP, IBCLC, CNE,
Rita F. D'Aoust, PhD, ANP-BC, CNE

KEYWORDS

- Accommodations • Civil rights • Disabilities • Inclusion • Nursing students
- Service animals • Universal design

KEY POINTS

- Nurses with disabilities add diversity to the profession, but many face multiple challenges in the work environment.
- The number of individuals with disabilities seeking admission to nursing school has increased.
- Although there are multiple challenges for students with disabilities (SWDs), students can disclose their disability and request accommodations at the time of admission or at any time in their nursing program.
- Considering the critical demand for nurses, technical standards should not exclude individuals with disabilities but should create a path by which nurses can be recruited.
- Creating reasonable accommodations for a student does not mean that the curriculum is revised for an individual.

INTRODUCTION

The introduction of the Americans with Disabilities Act (ADA) of 1990[1] protects civil rights and prohibits discrimination to individuals with physical and mental disabilities. Just as the ADA provides the commission of equal employment opportunities,[1] the act also ensures rights for equal access to educational opportunities for individuals with disabilities. Many nursing programs have previously used rigorous task statements as technical standards for admission, which did not relate to program outcomes.[2] Technical standards define the parameters of all that is needed to ensure safe and effective practice in nursing.[3] However, technical standards cannot specify how a skill

Johns Hopkins School of Nursing, 525 North Wolfe Street, Baltimore, MD 21205, USA
* Corresponding author.
E-mail address: llucas@jhmi.edu

Nurs Clin N Am 57 (2022) 671–683
https://doi.org/10.1016/j.cnur.2022.06.012
0029-6465/22/© 2022 Elsevier Inc. All rights reserved.
nursing.theclinics.com

will be accomplished, only that the person can accomplish the skill. Furthermore, although the nursing profession has endorsed the support of patients with disabilities, this support is not always reciprocated to nursing colleagues in the workplace.[4] This article reviews accommodations available for implementation in educational settings and describes environmental modifications and facilitative technologies for nursing students and nurses with disabilities.

The ADA defines disability as a physical or mental impairment that limits an individual's life activities.[1] Life activities are described as, for example, caring for oneself; performing manual tasks; and use of sensory skills and the ability to stand, walk, lift, bend, speak, breathe, learn, read, concentrate, think, and work.[1] Types of disabilities that may require accommodations include physical impairments such as visual and auditory limitations, chronic medical conditions with physical manifestations, emotional, psychiatric and mental health issues, and learning disabilities.[1,3]

Approximately 26% of the student population in higher education has a physical disability or experiences physical exacerbations manifested from chronic medical conditions.[2] The number of individuals with disabilities seeking admission to nursing school has increased in the last decade.[2,4,5] Consequently, the number of requests for accommodations has increased and is projected to continue to rise, leading to additional increases in nursing students who require accommodations.[2] A frequently cited faculty concern regarding students with disabilities (SWDs) is the stereotypical view that disabled students will not be able to provide safe care for their patients.[2,6]

Although there are multiple challenges for SWDs, students can disclose their disability and request accommodations at the time of admission or at any time during their nursing program. Accommodations in both the classroom and the clinical setting are permitted. Accommodations are assigned to an individual at the discretion of the institution's disability service.[2] Once approved, the challenge then becomes implementation of the accommodation for the student by the clinical and classroom faculty.

Failure to comply with the 2008 American With Disabilities Act Amendments Act[7] is violation of federal law.[4,6] Federal funding may be in jeopardy for programs, and fines may be imposed on institutions that do not comply with support for nursing SWDs. Those who believe they have not received the protection in accordance with their civil rights may file suit against an institution.

In the academic environment, it is the individual's responsibility to request and apply for accommodations. Self-advocacy skills need to be fostered in SWDs to facilitate communication of their needs regarding accommodations.[8] Neal-Boylan and colleagues[9,10] suggest that students use a mentor to assist with advocating for their rights. Students should work with the institution's accommodation officer to complete and submit documentation to obtain accommodations. Although it is the student's responsibility to decide when to share their accommodation with faculty, faculty prefer to have students to disclose their need for accommodations at the start of the semester to allow sufficient time for arranging and implementing plans,[4] especially for student accommodations in clinical areas. Accommodations are not required to be retroactive to the request, and time for faculty planning and collaboration is crucial to implementing accommodations for students.[2]

In addition to sufficient opportunity for planning, several other factors are key to providing effective accommodations. Flexibility for faculty in how they implement and use accommodations in a way that benefits the student is important.[2] For example, the requirement to arrive early for a day shift clinical may negatively impact the student's ability to function effectively due to the use of medication. Accommodations such as an evening shift clinical to support the student in their use of medication that makes it difficult for the student to arrive early may contribute to the student's success. Another example is the proximity of the clinical site to the student's home. A student who does not drive or has emotional stress with driving may request a clinical site that is close to the school or their home address. The student's positive attitude and professional demeanor regarding implementation of accommodations also contribute to their success.[2]

DEVICES AND ACCOMMODATIONS

Technical standards are defined as skills and abilities all nursing students should be able to demonstrate by the time they complete their academic program, but the way these skills should be performed or accomplished is not specified.[10] For disabled students, a need sometimes arises in a clinical area for the use of assistive devices, such as slings, braces, crutches, or devices to accommodate hearing or vision impairments that help students meet technical standards. Assistive devices may be required on a short- or long-term basis. Because patient and staff safety are a priority, hospital policies related to assistive devices must be followed.

Hearing Impairments

Individuals working in the medical profession may have a loss of higher frequency sounds or reverse-slope hearing loss, which refers to difficulty with hearing low-pitched frequency sounds.[11] Clear masks may be used by students with a hearing impairment so that lip reading (a technique of understanding speech by interpreting one's communication through visual observation of the mouth movements) can facilitate communication. Assistive technology such as an amplified stethoscope for hearing-impaired students can assist with assessing a blood pressure or auscultating lung, bowel, or heart sounds. Another option is an adaptive device for use with hearing aids. Depending on the type of hearing aid, and adjustment of the ear tips, a different form of ear tips may be useful.[11] If the student uses sign language, a sign language interpreter may also support learning in the classroom and in the clinical setting. It is important to understand that the interpreter is permitted to work for a limited number of hours, which may present a need for multiple interpreters during an 8-hour clinical day.

Visual Impairments

In a study exploring faculty perceptions of potential effects of different types of disabilities on student success, L'Ecuyer found that faculty were most concerned about nursing students with visual impairments.[12] Faculty attributed their concerns about nursing students with visual impairments to the need for accuracy in assessments, medication administration, and other interventions that depend on the student's ability to see. However, accommodations are available to support those with visual disabilities such as Braille or large-print textbooks and screen-reader technology. Scribes who can transfer test responses to required formats or record dictated notes and essays are also available. Learning technologies also allow use of specific colors, good color contrast, and larger font sizes that support general principles of universal design and usability.[13]

Service Animals

Just as there has been an increase in the number of students requesting accommodations in nursing school, there has also been an increase in the number of requests to use assistive animals in nursing programs.[14] It is important to note that only a service animal, defined as a dog that is specially trained to perform tasks for a person with a disability, will have protection under the ADA of 1990.[1] Service animals include animals trained to assist those who have visual impairment, diabetes, seizures, and post-traumatic stress disorder.[15] Assistance animals include service animals, therapy animals, and emotional support animals, and they may be used by nursing students for a range of conditions such as visual impairments, anxiety, seizures, and diabetes.[15]

It is important for faculty and administrators to understand federal, state, and institutional regulations governing the use of service animals. For example, service animals are permitted in areas open to the public; however, certain areas in a health care facility that may be restricted from public access include food preparation areas, operating rooms, intensive care units, sterile supply areas, isolation areas, and maternity units.[15] It is the responsibility of the institution to create a supportive learning experience for a student with a service animal. Once a student with a service animal has been admitted to the nursing program, communication with faculty, the clinical institution, and the clinical unit is vital in planning for the classroom and clinical experience.[15] If the student is comfortable disclosing information, one strategy to facilitate acceptance of the service animal by faculty, clinical preceptors, and peers is for the student to create a brief video that introduces the student and the service animal. This gives the student an opportunity to share information and introduce the dog to everyone who will interact with the student who uses the service animal. Information in the video should include directions to not interact, distract, or pet the dog, although it is working. If there are any staff or students who have allergies to dander, their schedules or assignment for the shift may need to be modified when the service animal is present in the clinical area. Guidelines for the clinical area should be established which address obtaining permission from the patient assigned to the student, identification of restricted areas where the service animal is not allowed, caring for the service animal during the shift, and planning for disposition of the service animal in the event of an emergency. Care for the service animal may include a cage, if appropriate, and a location and schedule for the service animal to take breaks.

Testing Accommodations

SWDs must be provided with equitable opportunities to demonstrate learning through accommodations related to testing and examinations.[16] The need for testing accommodations may be the result of multiple factors including anxiety, trouble with reading, being easily distracted, and slow thought processing speed.[17] Regardless of the factors involved, students must initiate the request for testing accommodations. Testing formats such as multiple choice questions, essay or short answer responses, use of mathematical computations, and paper/pencil versus computerized testing are variables to be considered when determining appropriate testing accommodations. Testing formats and related accommodations can be streamlined through the use of learning managements systems and other appropriate learning technologies. Best practices in online instructional design for all students require faculty to include vendor accessibility statements related to the learning management system and any other learning technologies used in the delivery of instruction.[18] Testing accommodations may include the use of extended testing time (time-and-a-half or double time), orally read directions, alterations in presentation (the use of large print or oral presentation), and a reduced-distraction environment. The use of extended time is the accommodation implemented most frequently,[17] with more than 90% of institutions using extended testing time for SWDs.[18] Although approximately one-third of students who request extended time as an accommodation (36%) do not use their extended time on examinations, faculty should still allow extra time as an accommodation because 64% of students use at least some portion of the extended time allowed to them, and simply having extended time available is enough to decrease student stress.[19] Although extended testing time may be effective for students, the impact of fatigue and potential overlap of examinations must be considered if a student is scheduled for multiple examinations with extended time.

For some students, the need to formulate thoughts and put them into legible or readable sentences to demonstrate knowledge is a challenge. Computer-based testing can take longer and be more difficult to follow for some SWDs. The student may need to reread sentences multiple times which can be distracting, increase their anxiety, and decrease their test performance. Student have identified specific challenges to seeking accommodations, including the process of scheduling their accommodated test date and time, not having instructor present to clarify questions or having an instructor who was not familiar with the provision of accommodations, and negative social implications when peers perceive an unfair advantage was conferred through testing accommodations.[17] Overall, students have reported positive benefits from extended time for examinations including less anxiety, improved grades, an equitable opportunity to demonstrate knowledge acquisition, and the sense of support from the faculty and the institution.[17]

Education about test-taking strategies may help all students, including those with and without identified disabilities. Although reviewing and test-taking strategies are not specifically identified as an accommodation, many students reported that they have never been taught about approaches to taking tests.[17] Test-taking strategies may include previewing the entire examination to identify how to allocate time effectively, spending limited time on an answer before moving on, backtracking if an answer cannot be determined on the first reading, writing down key points immediately, and eliminating answers with each question. Because the nursing licensure examination does not allow backtracking, many nursing schools do not allow students to backtrack on examination questions, which eliminate backtracking as a potential test-taking strategy. On the other hand, not allowing backtracking reduces the likelihood of second-guessing oneself and changing a correct answer to an incorrect answer.

Recommendations for testing accommodations include considerations for both policy and process. Faculty should be knowledgeable regarding the process for implementing accommodations. Utilization of the institution's student disabilities office is highly recommended, with one person assigned as the liaison for student and faculty interaction and planning. In addition, a clear policy regarding the process for students to receive their accommodation services and one team or one person whom students may contact to schedule examinations is recommended.

Course and Clinical Assignments

All students are held to the same expectations regarding course and clinical assignments, including students with approved accommodations, and receive appropriate documentation and feedback regarding missed clinical time and professional concerns. In the clinical area, accommodations may result in differences in the way clinical expectations are met, depending on the type of disability the student discloses. An accommodation does not give a student the option to do less than what is required from all students to accomplish the overall objectives of the course. The accommodation policies and processes ensure that the faculty will provide for approved accommodations consistently in a supportive environment. Accommodations may include a specific shift, such as evening shift or a nonrotating shift. In this case, clinical requirements could be met equitably on either a day or evening shift. Other accommodations may include having a chair to sit on at intervals, the need to take breaks, or an occasional late arrival to clinical. A physical device, if approved by the clinical site, may be used in an accommodation if it presents no safety concerns for the patient, students, or staff. In some cases, an accommodation may include not being in the same clinical group with another specific student if there has been conflict or tension between students in past courses or clinical experiences. This type of accommodation should be communicated to the appropriate faculty member.

Additional accommodations can be identified for both written and clinical assignments. For example, in a unique case, a student who had a disability that affected the ability to demonstrate knowledge acquisition on multiple choice tests was permitted to write a short answer response to the question prompts, and the faculty evaluated the accuracy of the response in alignment with the correct answer on the multiple choice examination. It is the responsibility of the student to make their particular needs known to appropriate individuals. This can be facilitated through a formal process in which the student participates or an informal process in which the student informs the appropriate individuals. For example, if the accommodation applies to theory courses and formal testing, the clinical faculty may not need to be informed. If the accommodation involves clinical participation, the theory faculty may not need to be informed.

Religious Accommodations

According to the Pew Research Center,[20] the United States is a religiously diverse country. Although most (89%) of those living in the United States identify as Christians who believe in God, there are rising numbers of those who identify with other religions.[20] Students may have religious traditions that are revered and practiced on an individual basis in conjunction with their beliefs, but there can be significant challenges to inclusion of those individuals in academic environments, and those challenges limit clinical opportunities for students and ultimately create gaps in the nursing workforce.[20] Nursing schools can promote opportunities for diversity in academic and clinical settings by providing accommodations for religious practices in the academic environment.

Religious accommodations include allowances for religious practices and observance of religious holidays. Although universities and nursing schools are commonly closed for many traditional Christian holidays, consideration should be given to approved absences for religious observances not included in a typical academic calendar. Nursing students may request accommodations for time off for a religious observance on a reoccurring or intermittent basis. An example of a reoccurring accommodation is a request for time to perform religious and spiritual practices such as daily prayers on a clinical day. Another reoccurring accommodation may be the need to leave the clinical area before sunset on Friday until sunset on Saturday.

Religious accommodations may also include dietary restrictions, dress requirements, grooming requirement (facial hair), and gender-concordant care. Although the acquisition of foods to support the cultural and religious traditions affiliated with practice is an individual responsibility, the accommodation may be in the form of support to have a meal or fast during a period of the day. Regarding dress and apparel, recognition of the meaning behind the attire is needed as well as the impact on patient care. For example, for those who practice covering their arms and wearing dresses as opposed to pants, faculty and administrators must review the institution's professional attire policy and make decisions about appropriate alternatives, if necessary. Another example is a head covering, or hijab, which is used to cover the head, ears, and neck for those who adhere to modest dress. Options that maintain alignment with best practices have been identified for the use of the hijab in the perioperative setting, which traditionally did not allow a hijab.[21] For students in a laboratory clinical experience such as health assessment, honoring requests for gender accommodations should be supported. Gender accommodations facilitate learning as each student can practice skills and assessments on a person with whom they are comfortable and in a setting that is supportive. Although the opportunity to offer gender accommodations is honored on patient request, the opportunity for nurses to request gender-concordant care is not yet a common practice (**Table 1**, for summary of accommodations).

RESOURCES

Although many schools of nursing have an affiliation with a large university that provides centralized disability services, smaller nursing schools may not have resources readily available to assist students with accommodations. Educators, academic partners, faculty, and nurses must be aware of the need for nursing students' accommodations and identify procedures to implement accommodations in all instructional settings. Education and information sharing is required to provide consistent support for those students with approved accommodations. As students graduate and seek

Table 1
Accommodations

Types of Accommodation	Recommendations and Devices
Assistive devices[10]	• Successful demonstration of skills and abilities is essential • Follow clinical agency policy regarding specific devices
Hearing impairment[11]	• Clear masks • Use of an interpreter • Use of an amplified stethoscope • Use of an adaptive device with hearing aids • Suggest adjustment of ear tips
Visual impairment[12]	• Assistive technology: screen reader, enlarged print (font size), font color
Service animals[14,15]	• Permitted in areas open to public, but certain areas are restricted in the clinical agency • Create a video to introduce service animal to staff • Modify staff schedules if fear/allergies are present • Identify plan for service animal in case of emergencies
Testing[16–19,22]	• Consider format (multiple choice, essay, short answer) • Time to take examination • Environment • Test-taking strategies
Assignments: class	• Extended deadlines • Identification of resources
Assignments: clinical	• Specific shift (AM/PM) • Proximity of institution (driving time) • Use of physical device • Availability of chair • Create specific assignments if there is a history of conflict between two or more individuals
Religious[21]	• Ability to be home before sundown on Sabbath • Time to practice religious and spiritual practices during clinical • Dress and grooming • Gender-concordant care • Support for dietary practices

employment, a supportive workplace environment with an atmosphere of understanding can have a positive impact on recruitment and retention of nurses who require accommodations. Identification of a specific staff member who will facilitate requests for accommodations and provide emotional, social, and psychological support throughout the process of securing accommodations can be helpful.[5,23]

EDUCATION
Regulatory Agencies and Competencies

National, state, and local regulatory agencies identify standards for nursing. The American Association of Colleges of Nursing (AACN) and the National Council of State Boards of Nursing (NCSBN) are two national regulatory nursing agencies that provide educational guidelines for nurses to perform with or without disabilities. The AACN[24] and NCSBN[25] have established essential functions that can be separated and categorized into cognitive, psychomotor, affective, and communication capabilities. The essential functions or standards provide competency guidelines for nursing programs to follow in design and implementation of instruction for students in classroom, laboratory, and clinical settings.[26] The state boards of nursing for each state, together with the AACN and NCSBN, hold academic nursing programs and individual nurses accountable for safe practice.

In addition to the guidelines from national and state agencies, there are *technical standards* for admission to nursing education. The technical standards are nonacademic requirements for admission to a nursing program and include important skills such as communication, critical thinking, attention to detail, and flexibility.[27] Although many consider the requirement to meet technical standards a barrier for individuals with disabilities, technical standards should not be confused with essential functions. Employers determine the *essential functions* for a particular job, which relate to each employment setting and specific job. Essential functions differ from technical standards in higher education, which define the parameters of what occurs to ensure safe and effective practice in a given field, such as the nursing profession. Technical standards cannot specify how a skill must be accomplished; they can only require that a person accomplish the skill. They must reflect current practice and not historic precedence.[3] For example, a standard might be that the individual must be able to detect blood pressure and heart sounds, but it cannot state that the individual must use specific equipment (such as a standard stethoscope and blood pressure cuff) to accomplish this. The use of nontraditional equipment would be a reasonable accommodation.[3]

Considering the critical demand for nurses, technical standards should not exclude those with disabilities but should create a path by which nurses can be recruited.[27] The path for recruitment would include nursing school policies which are inclusive of all individuals who are capable of learning about nursing and who will add to a diverse and qualified nursing workforce. Although all nursing students must rotate through various clinical experiences, individuals with disabilities and those needing accommodations will choose employment in a health care setting where they will be able to provide safe care and contribute to the nursing profession. The overarching goal for all stakeholders is to minimize barriers and maximize diversity in the nursing workforce.

Learning and Technology

Creating reasonable accommodations for a student does not mean that the curriculum is revised for an individual. A reasonable accommodation creates an opportunity for the student to succeed. Institutional policy must clearly identify student guidelines in terms of their program of study. For example, if a leave of absence is requested, the length of the leave and number of opportunities for a leave must be clearly defined. Other policies that may impact accommodations include course withdrawal, incomplete course work, criteria for passing a course, under what conditions a course must be repeated, and a minimum grade point average (GPA) to graduate. Courses with a clinical component must identify required clinical competencies and the impact of student performance in the clinical component on successful overall completion of the course.

Faculty should use creativity and continuous improvement processes in learning design to encourage engagement for all students and support comprehension of content. Examples of accessible digital course activities include videos, unfolding case studies, group learning or team-based activities, and voice-over PowerPoint presentations, which provide flexible access to engaging ways to interact with peers and course content for all students. An interactive discussion forum application such as VoiceThread or Flipgrid transforms ordinary online text-based discussions into collaborative interactions using video and audio. Learning technologies such as Kaltura, Zoom, and Panopto can be used to record lectures and auto-generate closed captions. Although auto-generated closed captioning features in webinar and lecture capture applications are continually improving, it is important to note potential differences in accuracy between machine-generated and human-generated captions. Although machine-generated captions are time- and cost-efficient and immediately readable, they may be less accurate than human-generated captions, which tend to be very accurate but very costly and take longer to produce. However, students who disclose a hearing impairment may require human-generated or human-edited captions, if machine-generated captions are not sufficiently accurate. Good microphone equipment, optimal audio conditions, and limiting speakers to one person who can talk at a time improve.

Virtual meeting spaces such as Zoom, Skype, and MicrosoftTeams are online applications with a variety of accessibility features that can be used to promote student interaction in a group setting when social distancing and the opportunity for in-person meetings are limited. Virtual simulation technology provides students with clinical simulation opportunities, including telehealth simulations, that can be conducted online any time and in any place that has a connection to the Internet. Virtual reality and augmented reality offer a unique simulation experience facilitated by individual headgear for visual and audio use, although the implications of using virtual reality hardware and software in teaching SWDs are not yet well understood. It is important to remember to make accessibility statements from software vendors available to all students when any learning technology is used to deliver content or implement instructional experiences.

Faculty

Although it is the student's responsibility to initiate communication regarding the need for accommodations, the faculty also have educational needs and responsibilities related to teaching SWDs. Nursing schools need to establish policies and procedures that provide education and support for faculty regarding teaching SWDs and faculty responsibilities in response to a student's request for accommodations. First, the request for accommodations should be reasonable and comply with the ADA.[10] The policies should include supportive information regarding the person or department the student must contact to establish the need for an accommodation; the flow of communication to the faculty, including how information will be shared; and the person responsible for meeting with the student to establish a plan and follow-up on the progress of the student. Policies should not be so rigid that they create a barrier to individuals with disabilities, nor should the accommodations be so lax as to interfere with fundamental components of the academic program. An example of a policy that is too lax would be permitting a student to create their own part-time plan of study when a fundamental component of the program is a full-time curriculum in which clinical courses are sequential to promote logical progression of learning. Having a designated individual at the institution or nursing school that has specialized knowledge of accommodations, processes, legal ramifications, and ways to support students and faculty will help keep policies and processes reasonable for all stakeholders and in alignment with the ADA.

There is a strong need for cohesiveness in preparing to deal with accommodation requests, which includes communication between the student and the faculty. Although it is appropriate for faculty to focus on patient safety, medical errors are typically caused by systems, processes, or conditions that are faulty, as opposed to recklessness or characteristics of an individual.[26] Once the student has shared information regarding their request for accommodations for class or clinical, faculty members will need to provide the necessary support. If the accommodation request will impact the clinical experience, planning and collaboration with the partner institution will be needed with clear communication between clinical coordinators and specific faculty members. Program directors are responsible for ensuring appropriate policies are in place to provide guidance to the faculty for student support and success and support the student's successful completion of the program.

NURSING EMPLOYMENT AFTER GRADUATION
Clinical Environment

Nursing students who require accommodations will graduate and seek employment as nurses. Many nurses fail to disclose the need for accommodations due to fear of not being accepted or being subjected to discrimination in the workplace. They also worry that they will not be hired or will lose their job. Many nurses with disabilities have expressed that their experience in nursing school was a way to prove themselves worthy of being a nurse.[10] Nurses with disabilities have also identified the misconception that disability is associated with a lack of intelligence or the ability to understand. According to Neal-Boylan and Miller,[10] nurses with disabilities are very successful in their profession and attribute their ability to be more empathetic as a nurse to their experience in their nursing programs.

The Office of Federal Contract Compliance Programs (OFCCP) is a government agency that protects workers from discrimination and enforces the law while promoting diversity.[28] Specifically, Section 503 of the Rehabilitation Act of 1973 prohibits federal contractors and subcontractors from discriminating against individuals with disabilities.[29] The OFCCP encourages those with disabilities to voluntarily self-identify as a way to create and support change as well as assist with equal employment opportunities.

Patients' Rights

Ultimately, patients always have the right to refuse care from the nurse who has been assigned to them. Although patients may see noticeable disabilities in their nurse, it does not mean that their nurse is any less competent or not able to provide safe and efficient care. Nurses with disabilities have more empathy for their patients compared with those who have no disabilities.[10] In addition, nurses work in a variety of settings in which they perform various essential functions. Nurses must safely accomplish certain skills in specific clinical settings, and *how* they go about accomplishing a specific skill is not necessarily the focus.[10]

SUMMARY

As the profession of nursing continues to embrace principles of diversity, equity, and inclusion, support for the success of nursing students and nurses with disabilities is crucial in academics and the workplace. There are opportunities for all stakeholders in nursing education to learn from nurses and students regarding disabilities, and SWDs inspire educational innovation in nursing education and diversify the nursing workforce. It is also important to remember that a nurse may develop or identify a disability at any time during their career and especially as the nursing workforce ages. Inclusion and support for nurses with disabilities is of utmost importance to the profession.

The development of academic and clinical best practices for inclusion of nurses and nursing SWDs must be a collaborative effort among nursing schools, clinical partners, and patient settings. Acknowledging a need to improve diversity by providing accommodations to those who need them is an important first step, but education and policy changes are vital. In light of the expanding critical need for nurses, the profession of nursing is poised to enhance the culture of education, understanding, acceptance, tolerance, and inclusion around nursing students and nurses with accommodations for disabilities. Improvements in policy and practice related to accommodations for disabilities will lead to increased recruitment and improved retention of nurses and contribute to better patient outcomes.

CLINICS CARE POINTS

- Civil rights are protected and discrimination to individuals with physical and mental disabilities is prohibited under the Americans with Disabilities Act of 1990.
- Failure to comply with the 2008 American with Disabilities Act Amendments Act[7] is violation of federal law which could result in loss of federal funding.
- Online and digital resources, software, and hardware that meet accessibility and usability standards can improve learning experiences for all students.
- Assistive devices, learning technologies, service animals, and faculty familiarity with policies and procedures facilitate accommodations for students with disabilities.
- The development of accommodation policies and practices in the clinical and academic settings must be a collaborative effort among nursing schools, clinical partners, and patient-care settings.

DISCLOSURE

The authors have nothing to disclose.

REFERENCES

1. Americans with Disabilities Act of 1990. ADA.gov. Published June 15, 2009. Available at: https://www.ada.gov/pubs/adastatute08.htm#12111. Accessed December 1, 2021.

2. Horkey E. Reasonable academic accommodation implementation in clinical nursing education. Nurs Educ Perspect 2019;40(4):1.
3. Matt SB, Maheady D, Fleming SE. Educating nursing students with disabilities: Replacing essential functions with technical standards for program entry criteria. J Postsecondary Education Disabil 2015;28(4):461–8.
4. Neal-Boylan L, Smith D. Nursing students with physical disabilities: Dispelling myths and correcting misconceptions. Nurse Educ 2016;41(1):13–8.
5. Costello-Harris V. Evidence of inclusion on college websites: Academic accommodations and human support. J Postsecondary Education Disabil 2019;32(3): 263–78.
6. Davidson P, Rushton C, Dotzenrod J, et al. Just and realistic expectations for persons with disabilities practicing nursing. AMA J Ethics 2016;18(10):1034–40.
7. Americans with Disabilities Act Amendments Act of 2008. U.S. Equal Employment Opportunity Commission. 2021. Available at: https://www.eeoc.gov/statutes/americans-disabilities-act-amendments-act-2008. Accessed December 6, 2021.
8. Lindsay S, Cagliostro E, Leck J, et al. Career aspirations and workplace expectations among youth with physical disabilities. Disabil Rehabil 2019;43(12): 1657–68.
9. Marks B, McCulloh K. Success for students and nurses with disabilities. Nurse Educ 2016;41(1):9–12.
10. Neal-Boylan L, Miller M. Treat me like everyone else. Nurse Educ 2017;42(4): 176–80.
11. Clason D. Amplified stethoscopes assist healthcare workers who have hearing loss. Available at: https://www.healthyhearing.com/report/46018-Stethoscope-hearing-aids. Accessed December 2, 2021.
12. L'Ecuyer KM. Perceptions of nurse preceptors of students and new graduates with learning difficulties and their willingness to precept them in clinical practice (Part 2). Nurse Educ Pract 2019;34:210–7.
13. Henry SL, Abou-Zahra S, White K. Accessibilty, usability, and inclusion. Retrieved on February 12, 2022. Available at: https://www.w3.org/WAI/fundamentals/accessibility-usability-inclusion/. Accessed December 29, 2021.
14. Shilling S, Lucas L, Silbert-Flagg J, et al. Federal, state, and institutional regulations regarding a nursing student with a service animal. J Prof Nurs 2020;36(6): 454–7.
15. Silbert-Flagg J, Shilling SD, Lucas L, et al. Preparing for a student with a service animal. J Prof Nurs 2020;36(6):458–61.
16. Greenberg D. Technical Report: Overview of disability law for higher education, National Center for College Students with Disabilities, 2017.
17. Slaughter MH, Lindstrom JH, Anderson R. Perceptions of extended time accommodations among postsecondary students with disabilities. Exceptionality 2020;1–15. https://doi.org/10.1080/09362835.2020.1727339.
18. QM Rubric (2020). Available at: https://www.qualitymatters.org/sites/default/files/PDFs/QM-Higher-Ed-Sixth-Edition-Specific-Review-Standards-Accessible.pdf. Accessed February 13, 2022.
19. Sokal L, Vermette L. Double time? Examining extended testing time accommodations (ETTA) in postsecondary settings. J Postsecondary Education Disabil 2017; 30(2):185–200.
20. Pew Research Center. U.S. public becoming less religious. Available at: http://assets.pewresearch.org/wp-content/uploads/sites/11/2015/11/201.11.03_RLS_II_full_report.pdf. Accessed December 29, 2021.

21. Hopkins AF, Kooken WC, Winger EN. Inclusive clinical practice and policy for Muslim nursing students. J Transcult Nurs 2019;31(1):100–6.
22. Raue K, Lewis L. Students with disabilities at degree-granting postsecondary institutions. National Center for Education Statistics; 2011. Available at: https://eric.ed.gov/?id=ED520976.
23. Barrett M. Working with students with disabilities at the SON. Address presented at the Johns Hopkins School of Nursing, November 17, 2021.
24. The Essentials of Baccalaureate Education for Professional Nursing Practice October 20, 2008. American Association of Colleges of Nursing (AACN). Available at: https://www.aacnnursing.org/portals/42/publications/baccessentials08.pdf. Accessed December 5, 2021.
25. National Council of State Boards of Nursing 1996. NCSBN. Available at: https://www.ncsbn.org/1996_Part1.pdf. Accessed December 5, 2021.
26. Yarbrough A, *Discovering the Process of Reasonable Academic Accommodations for Pre-licensure Nursing Students with Learning Disabilities, 2019, Doctoral dissertation*, University of Georgia.
27. Ailey SH, Marks B. Technical standards for nursing education programs in the 21st century. Rehabil Nurs 2020;45(6):311–20.
28. Office of Federal Contract Compliance Programs (OFCCP). U.S. Department of Labor, Office of Federal Contract Compliance Programs. Available at: https://www.dol.gov/agencies/ofccp. Accessed December 5, 2021.
29. Bruyère S.M., Employment and disability: issues, innovations, and opportunities, *Labor And Employment Relations Association*, 2020, Cornell University Press.

UNITED STATES POSTAL SERVICE ®

Statement of Ownership, Management, and Circulation
(All Periodicals Publications Except Requester Publications)

1. Publication Title	2. Publication Number	3. Filing Date
NURSING CLINICS OF NORTH AMERICA	598 – 960	9/18/2022

4. Issue Frequency	5. Number of Issues Published Annually	6. Annual Subscription Price
MAR, JUN, SEP, DEC	4	$163

7. Complete Mailing Address of Known Office of Publication (Not printer) (Street, city, county, state, and ZIP+4®)

ELSEVIER INC.
230 Park Avenue, Suite 800
New York, NY 10169

Contact Person
Malathi Samayan

Telephone (Include area code)
91-44-4299-4507

8. Complete Mailing Address of Headquarters or General Business Office of Publisher (Not printer)

ELSEVIER INC.
230 Park Avenue, Suite 800
New York, NY 10169

9. Full Names and Complete Mailing Addresses of Publisher, Editor, and Managing Editor (Do not leave blank)

Publisher (Name and complete mailing address)

DOLORES MELONI, ELSEVIER INC.
1600 JOHN F KENNEDY BLVD. SUITE 1800
PHILADELPHIA, PA 19103-2899

Editor (Name and complete mailing address)

KERRY HOLLAND, ELSEVIER INC.
1600 JOHN F KENNEDY BLVD. SUITE 1800
PHILADELPHIA, PA 19103-2899

Managing Editor (Name and complete mailing address)

PATRICK MANLEY, ELSEVIER INC.
1600 JOHN F KENNEDY BLVD. SUITE 1800
PHILADELPHIA, PA 19103-2899

10. Owner (Do not leave blank. If the publication is owned by a corporation, give the name and address of the corporation immediately followed by the names and addresses of all stockholders owning or holding 1 percent or more of the total amount of stock. If not owned by a corporation, give the names and addresses of the individual owners. If owned by a partnership or other unincorporated firm, give its name and address as well as those of each individual owner. If the publication is published by a nonprofit organization, give its name and address.)

Full Name	Complete Mailing Address
WHOLLY OWNED SUBSIDIARY OF REED/ELSEVIER, US HOLDINGS	1600 JOHN F KENNEDY BLVD. SUITE 1800 PHILADELPHIA, PA 19103-2899

11. Known Bondholders, Mortgagees, and Other Security Holders Owning or Holding 1 Percent or More of Total Amount of Bonds, Mortgages, or Other Securities. If none, check box ☑ None

Full Name	Complete Mailing Address
N/A	

12. Tax Status (For completion by nonprofit organizations authorized to mail at nonprofit rates) (Check one)
The purpose, function, and nonprofit status of this organization and the exempt status for federal income tax purposes:
☑ Has Not Changed During Preceding 12 Months
☐ Has Changed During Preceding 12 Months (Publisher must submit explanation of change with this statement)

PS Form **3526**, July 2014 [Page 1 of 4 (see instructions page 4)]   PSN: 7530-01-000-9931   PRIVACY NOTICE: See our privacy policy on www.usps.com.

13. Publication Title		14. Issue Date for Circulation Data Below
NURSING CLINICS OF NORTH AMERICA		JUNE 2022

15. Extent and Nature of Circulation			Average No. Copies Each Issue During Preceding 12 Months	No. Copies of Single Issue Published Nearest to Filing Date
a. Total Number of Copies (Net press run)			401	335
b. Paid Circulation (By Mail and Outside the Mail)	(1)	Mailed Outside-County Paid Subscriptions Stated on PS Form 3541 (Include paid distribution above nominal rate, advertiser's proof copies, and exchange copies)	281	230
	(2)	Mailed In-County Paid Subscriptions Stated on PS Form 3541 (Include paid distribution above nominal rate, advertiser's proof copies, and exchange copies)	0	0
	(3)	Paid Distribution Outside the Mails Including Sales Through Dealers and Carriers, Street Vendors, Counter Sales, and Other Paid Distribution Outside USPS®	83	75
	(4)	Paid Distribution by Other Classes of Mail Through the USPS (e.g. First-Class Mail®)	0	0
c. Total Paid Distribution (Sum of 15b (1), (2), (3), and (4))			364	305
d. Free or Nominal Rate Distribution (By Mail and Outside the Mail)	(1)	Free or Nominal Rate Outside-County Copies included on PS Form 3541	37	30
	(2)	Free or Nominal Rate In-County Copies Included on PS Form 3541	0	0
	(3)	Free or Nominal Rate Copies Mailed at Other Classes Through the USPS (e.g. First-Class Mail)	0	0
	(4)	Free or Nominal Rate Distribution Outside the Mail (Carriers or other means)	0	0
e. Total Free or Nominal Rate Distribution (Sum of 15d (1), (2), (3) and (4))			37	30
f. Total Distribution (Sum of 15c and 15e)			401	335
g. Copies not Distributed (See Instructions to Publishers #4 (page #3))			0	0
h. Total (Sum of 15f and g)			401	335
i. Percent Paid (15c divided by 15f times 100)			90.77%	91.04%

* If you are claiming electronic copies, go to line 16 on page 3. If you are not claiming electronic copies, skip to line 17 on page 3.

16. Electronic Copy Circulation	Average No. Copies Each Issue During Preceding 12 Months	No. Copies of Single Issue Published Nearest to Filing Date
a. Paid Electronic Copies ▶		
b. Total Paid Print Copies (Line 15c) + Paid Electronic Copies (Line 16a) ▶		
c. Total Print Distribution (Line 15f) + Paid Electronic Copies (Line 16a) ▶		
d. Percent Paid (Both Print & Electronic Copies) (16b divided by 16c × 100) ▶		

☑ I certify that 50% of all my distributed copies (electronic and print) are paid above a nominal price.

17. Publication of Statement of Ownership

☑ If the publication is a general publication, publication of this statement is required. Will be printed
in the DECEMBER 2022 issue of this publication.

☐ Publication not required.

18. Signature and Title of Editor, Publisher, Business Manager, or Owner

Malathi Samayan

Malathi Samayan - Distribution Controller

Date 9/18/2022

I certify that all information furnished on this form is true and complete. I understand that anyone who furnishes false or misleading information on this form or who omits material or information requested on the form may be subject to criminal sanctions (including fines and imprisonment) and/or civil sanctions (including civil penalties).

PS Form **3526**, July 2014 (Page 3 of 4)   PRIVACY NOTICE: See our privacy policy on www.usps.com.

Printed and bound by CPI Group (UK) Ltd, Croydon, CR0 4YY

03/10/2024

01040469-0019